Possibly The Greatest Weight Control Breakthrough Of The Century

WEIGHT CONTROL BREAKTHROUGH IS NEXT ARTICLE DOWN:
ALL MINIMUM WAGE LAWS MUST BE BANNED IF WESTERN CIVILIZATION IS TO SURVIVE, PERIOD.

SURE, AN EPIC DEATH BATTLE TO SAVE WESTERN CIVILIZATION IS GOING DOWN. BUT, THE BATTLE IS NOT WHAT ALMOST EVERYONE THANKS IT IS. THE REAL BATTLE IS CONSERVATISM VERSUS LIBERALISM AND IGNORANCE, WITH LIBERALISM ALREADY HAVING TAKEN OVER DAMN NEAR EVERYTHING.

LIBERALISM AND IGNORANCE IS THE TRUE IDEOLOGY THAT HAS AND WILL FINISH DESTROYING WESTERN CIVILIZATION UNLESS DRASTIC ACTION IS TAKEN SOON.

ONLY BANNING ALL MINIMUM WAGE LAWS CAN SAVE WESTERN CIVILIZATION BEFORE IT COMPLETELY SELF-DESTRUCTS DUE TO LIBERALISM AND IGNORANCE. SURE, ALL OF THIS OTHER STUFF MATTERS BUT FIRST THINGS FIRST.

ABORTION: THE RICH HAS ALWAYS MURDERED FUTURE UNBORN BABIES IN THE WOMB, BUT NEVER HAS THE POOR MASS MURDERED IN THE WOMB UNTIL AFTER OUR "NEW DEAL" WELFARE STATE. IT IS A CRIME AGAINST NATURE NO MATTER HOW ONE LOOKS AT IT.

ANYONE THAT KNOWINGLY AND INTENTIONALLY MURDERS FUTURE UNBORN BABIES IN THE WOMB PAYS WITH OVER POWERING GUILT, OR DEVELOPS CONTEMPT FOR HUMAN LIFE ITSELF TO AVOID GOING INSANE. (ISMDH).

POSSIBLY THE GREATEST WEIGHT CONTROL BREAKTHROUGH OF THE CENTURY:

1

Possibly The Greatest Weight Control Breakthrough Of The Century

95 percent of losing weight is mental in my view. I decided to offer this as a bonus, hope you find it useful. Freddie L Sirmans' weight losing helpful hint using the "Positive thinking" technique. The definition of the positive thinking technique I'm talking about is: One takes a short saying or quote and repeats it over and over to ones self a minimum of fifty times or more every day.

It may take up to six months or more to start feeling strong results. This is the quote I use: "I can keep my body slim and healthy through God which strengthens me." Just leave God off or substitute another deity if one doesn't believe in God.

Lets face it folks, some of us like me are compulsive over eaters; I have suffered with this disorder ever since I was a child. Some of us just simply can't do it alone that is why turning to God by saying through God, which strengthens me, is all-powerful.

However, it doesn't work over night, it takes a while to break through to the subconscious. But, if one stays the course long enough positive results will be realized.

Be aware, the mind tries all kinds of tricks to throw one off his/her game. After saying the quote awhile one may crave to eat more and feel it is a waste of time so why bother. So, I just stayed the course and refuse to give up.

THE NEXT FIVE ARTICLES DOWN ARE MY OLDER MUST READ ARTICLES:

THE FOLLY OF THINKING THE USA BUDGET CAN BE BALANCED?

A genuine true non-phony free market place economy without exception must be able to set its own wages and prices, period. The liberals in charge of the government seized that right when they enacted the evil 1938 socialist minimum wage law.

That act castrated the USA economy and has led to the destruction of our culture and morals. And until the USA economy is given back its power by repealing the evil 1938 socialist minimum wage law nothing can break the liberals choke hold on this great nation. Otherwise, there is simply no way this great nation of individual freedom can ever be saved.

Men and women of sound mind with strong survival instincts must give the USA economy back its true power, that way it can save this great nation. Nothing else has the power and discipline to drain this vast liberal swamp and prevent individual freedom from disappearing off the face of the earth forever. God save the USA the last bastion of true individual freedom left in the world today.

The truth of the matter is government is actually a parasite; it can only survive if it has a host to take from. Government is not part of the economy but what it does greatly affects the economy. Every society must have a means of protecting itself from internal and external threats and dangers, and that makes having some form of government a must.

Most governments have the power to take over that is why most private sector host has strong built in protections and total control over the money supply. But, like they say, "The way to hell is paved with good intentions."

On the surface the government doing good and helping people doesn't seem like a threat, and it is not in perspective on a temporary basis. But, in reality government must never become a social and family provider more than on a temporary basis if a free nation is to survive long term.

Whoever is the provider is the boss like it or not. That is why in the USA and Western Europe for all practical purpose the welfare state has taken over. Today there are far too many people dependent on the government to ever put government spending on a diet.

In Western Europe and now in the USA the money priority first goes to the welfare state over the military and all else. And there is only contempt for the profit driven private business enterprise host. Plus, private business days may be numbers because liberal media and the masses don't understand profit and hate it.

Still, there is a savior waiting on a white horse ready to ride in to rescue western civilization. But first, the evil 1938 socialist minimum law must be shot with a silver bullet or a stake driven through its heart by repealing or getting rid of all minimum wage laws entirely. This evil poison pill law must be buried to never rise again for any democracy to ever be safe.

In terms of raw bare boned survival using good intentions and doing the right thing may cause Mother Nature to spit in your face. Just look at the animal

kingdom with raw nature, there is no place for good
intentions or doing the right thing, except to starve.

Now, you look at the USA economic situation, from a
political point of view good intentions and doing the
right thing I believe will surely get you booted out of
power, period. Folks, let me stop right here and
explain, I'm a writer and I write it as I see it. I can be
wrong, in fact I hope I am wrong on some of the dire
things I see coming down the pike.

I have said it before and am going to say it again,
anyone that still thinks the USA and western Europe
can be saved as welfare states is economically ignorant
in my view. Maybe I'm the one who is ignorant.
However, I believe I can dissect and understand the
inner workings of an economy as well as anyone.

Yet, for the life of me I can't see any social and family
provider welfare state doing anything but slowly
devouring its own survival host, which is private
business enterprise. Economically, it is just impossible
for a welfare state to survive very much longer by
constantly dwindling its own only survival host, which
is profit driven private business enterprise.

Government can take only so much profit before there
is none left to take. Anyone with common sense should
know that the USA can't forever reckless spend and
keep going deeper and deeper into debt. A reasonable
person should conclude that the right thing to do is
balance the budget and get your physical house in
order.

Possibly The Greatest Weight Control Breakthrough Of The Century

Sure, that is the responsible thing to do if you are talking about around 80 years ago right after the minimum wage law was enacted. But, today for a political party to take that type of normal responsible action is political suicide.

Now, here is where my super wisdom comes into play. OK, lets just imagine that at the snap of fingers all of the USA debts are paid free and clear, do you think the health of the nation would be solved? My answer would be no! Our debt is a currency problem but civilization existed long before a currency was invented.

The main problems with the USA and western civilization are culture and moral in my view. Contrary to the common view I believe in free nations the economy is the real disciplinarian that actually guards and protects the nations culture and morals.

Sure, we are a nation ruled by law not by man, but I believe the economy is the real power that pulls the strings behind the scene. Also, I believe liberalism is actually what's destroying the USA, which could never have happen with a genuine true free market place economy.

I feel the economy the USA has today is a phony P.... of an economy and has been that way ever since the evil 1938 minimum wage law was enacted. The economy the USA has today doesn't have the power or discipline to protect itself or the nation's culture and morals.

Possibly The Greatest Weight Control Breakthrough Of The Century

Once the 1938 minimum wage law was enacted, that allowed liberalism a foot in the door to inflate the currency and grow government to no end. Since then the minimum wage law gave government absolute power over prices and wages. Once that happened the aggressive liberals has played to the basic weaknesses in our human nature by promising the moon and back.

The minimum wage law gave government complete control over private property rights and private business enterprise, which it had never had before in the history of the country. By repealing the minimum wage law the economy would regain its power to guard and protect the nations culture and morals, plus boom the economy in real growth not any phony inflated growth like today.

So, the republican think they can take on our welfare state beast and balance the budget, plus remain in power. Well, I'm one that thinks they are in for a very rude awakening. I hope I'm wrong, but I think the beast will defend itself and win. I truly feel only a genuine true free market place economy minus any minimum wage law has the power and ability to take down this beast.

They will never agree with me, but I feel the only wise course the republicans has left to save the USA is to repeal the evil 1938 socialist minimum wage law, "That is all she wrote." As to liberals saving the country, they are the ones hell bent on destroying it and too shallow to even realize it.

SIRMANS LOG: 17 MARCH 2015, 1748 HOURS.

OBEDIENCE OF THE LAW MUST BE THE FIRST PRIORITY, FAILURE TO DO SO LEAVES NO EXCUSE FOR WHATEVER MAY HAPPEN
We all care about our loved ones. But, the only thing that keeps us from behaving like wild animals in the jungle is the law. The law must be above all else and the top priority for the USA to remain a civilized nation.

The law must be respected and obeyed, period. We now have the law flaunted and disrespected in high places, and after years of our liberal entitlement welfare state many have succumbed to raw subjective emotionalism. Whatever happened to the words "No one is above the law," are they still valid?

You may want to be weak and stupid and live by the rules of the jungle with little or no respect for the law then have at it, just don't include me. I believe in "First things first," period. The law is what protects us all, especially the poor and disadvantage.

Part of what's wrong with this entitlement welfare state now is we have turned into a P…. society with less and less accountability. And it's going to be our downfall, you mark my word. Anyone that succumbs to the weakness of subjective emotionalism is a fool and loser, and is either ignorant or not dealing with a full deck in my view.

If one doesn't love and support unconditional one's own race he is without a true identity and can't really be trusted. It's a fact we African Americans are without a true identity and is searching for love in all of the wrong places. I've heard the chant, black and proud and all of that, but in my view it is just words and lack substance.

We need to believe we as African Americans are as
good as any race and need to take pride in behaving
and obeying the law as well as any race. If you want to
be treated with respect, then act like one deserving
respect. I believe we as a race can behave and obey
the law as well as any race, and we as a race did too
before our liberal entitlement welfare state came
about.

SIRMANS LOG: 04 DECEMBER 2014, 1658 HOURS

**WE AFRICAN AMERICANS HAS A PRIMITIVE
HERD MENTALITY WITH VERY LITTLE FREE
INDEPENDENT ACCOUNTABILITY THINKING
AMONG US:**
Most African Americans have a bond to the democrat
party like a child to its mother. And no amount of
reasoning or logic can break that bond unless the child
becomes a free independent minded thinker. Natures
law of "taking the course of least resistance" dictates
that almost no one is going to become a free
independent accountability thinker unless forced to.

The herd won't allow free independent accountability
thinking within the herd itself and even when an
individual does it anyway he is branded a traitor or nut
case. Hell, I love my country the only home I know
and I feel if you are wrong you deserve to be called
out even if you are a sister, brother, or mother.

I don't believe in pampering anyone, you are
responsible for your own actions. To err is human, and
forgiveness is the foundation of the Christian religion in
my view. I'm one that believes that civilization would
never have gotten out of the Dark Age without the
Christian religion and its power of forgiveness.

My God, I watch the local news almost everyday and

its smash and grab, armed robbery, breaking and interring, muggings, and crime galore. And guess who is doing almost all of this crime? You fill in the blank. Yet, all I hear from white liberals and black liberals is patronizing and misplaced guilt and no accountability what so ever, it's insane.

Before the "New deal" a trip behind the shed or woodpile would always keep the would be future criminals on the straight and narrow good citizen course and out of prison. Since that's not done very much any more the best thing that would do the most good for young future black criminals would be medical supervised flogging.

Four or five hard lick on the ass would do far more good than 5-10 in the pen and it wouldn't cost the tax payers. That would put a stop to this paying to produce a more harden and cunning criminal. But, that will never happen, oh, no, we are too civilized for that, yet, the cancer of crime is splitting this great country into racial camps, duh.

Only one thing can save the great USA now: repeal the cruel evil 1938 socialist minimum wage law, then there will be no government forced wage control. That would get rid of any forced wage control entirely. That is the only way this great nation can be saved from itself, period. Repeal it now tomorrow may be too late.
SIRMANS LOG: 30 NOVEMBER 2014, 2123 HOURS

INJECTION: 02 DECEMBER 2014, 1232 HOURS
A huge disadvantage with African Americans having a herd mentality is it has allows a very few poverty pimps to exploit and keep alive this still-a-victim big, big, big, lie. And as long as we have our liberal induced welfare state I see very little chance of African Americans ever being forced to take responsibility and stand on their own to gain a do-and-think-for -yourself

mentality.

Sure, I may be hated for my views now, but there will come a day when I will be loved for my great wisdom and foresight, glory be to God.

Just look at our African American situation, in some neighborhoods there is not a husband to be found for miles. And even if you can find a man living in some of the homes all he is there for is companionship and stud service at her whim. Uncle Sam is the real sugar daddy, a poor man can't compete. Come on y'all give me a break now, instead of all of this rioting we as a race ought to be cleaning up our own house.

We ought to be instilling in our young discipline and self-respect and respect for other people and their property, too. Shame on us for not knowing how to behave and obey the law like other races does. Other races have eyes; they see who is committing all of these crimes. Reality is reality, don't insult my intelligence.

Sure, we as race are guilty of keeping a child's mentality including a fierce sibling rivalry against those who look like us. That is why African Americans can't advance as a race; we won't readily support each other in business or otherwise unless there is no other good choice. And even our elites will try to get as far away from an all black neighborhood as they can afford.

All other races create different pecking order level surrounding zones in their own race's community, lets face facts, and it takes an independent minded adult to escape childhood sibling rivalry. And the first thing it takes to do that is the ability to forgive all people. Otherwise, un-forgiveness locks one in to that situation, then if one is still hating and un-forgiving seventy years later they will still have that fierce dependent minded sibling rivalry from childhood.

11

Possibly The Greatest Weight Control Breakthrough Of The Century

To escape here is a simple formula to repeat to yourself over and over until you mean it: "I can wish all people goodwill (through God who strengthens me), optional if you are a Christian." That will free one to become an independent thinker.

I never intended to get sidetracked off into all of this theory stuff, it seems as if my pen took on a life of its own, sorry. Sure, we as a race have some guilt in my view, but again the real arch villain behind the scene is the heavy hand of our liberal induced welfare state beast pulling the strings.

However, before the new deal African Americans had almost thrown off their dependency minded slave mentality, but the welfare state nipped all of that in the bud. Before the new deal blacks supported each other, and we had poor, middle class, and upper class zones in the same community. Plus, we had far more black owned businesses than today. Every town had a booming chitlin's circuit and great entertainment.

We were about to become of age. But, the New deal kicked the poor black man out of the house. After that no one instilled discipline, proper norms, and traditions in our young and we lost our way. After all of that our dependency minded slave mentality returned with a vengeance and the democrat party and the welfare state is now our new slave masters.
SIRMANS LOG: 02 DECEMBER 2014, 1232 HOURS

FERGUSON IS A WAKE-UP CALL ON WHAT CULTURE ROT AND MORAL DECAY HAS DONE TO THE USA DUE TO OUR LIBERAL INDUCED WELFARE STATE
NEW INJECTION #2, 25 NOVEMBER 2014, 1907 HOURS
What we African Americans need to realize is each of

12

us is an ambassador for our race. Many years ago we blacks knew that, but that seems to be lost now a days. A good or bad stereotype image affects all of us in some way, you can't escape it.

Call it what you may but there is no denying the fact that African Americans are committing far more crimes than any race on earth proportional-wise. The main reason for that is lack of parents instilling self-restraint and self-accountability in their young. A lack of self-restraint and self-accountability breeds disrespect for authority and the rights of others.

That is what's driving this out of control cancer in the African American community call crime. But, the actual real villain driving everything from behind the curtain is our liberal induced welfare state beast, with the ability to throw a rock and hide its hand. I stand by my prediction that the USA economy will collapse in 2015 unless our cruel evil 1938 socialist minimum wage law is repealed.

I see all of the economically ignorant do-gooders believing that raising the minimum wage will help people, but, in reality it will only speed up our pace to an economy collapsing doom. Getting rid of any wage or price control entirely is our only way out, because that will restore power back to the people then the people will need very little money and live off the land if need to.

However, there has never been a case of government changing course knowing it is headed to doom, it is not in its DNA. The powers that be is going to feed this tax hungry gobbling welfare state beast to the last crumb.

They will never stop feeding the beast and I will never stop drum beating to repeal our evil 1938 socialist minimum wage law to save the only home and way of life I know. Glory be to God.

Possibly The Greatest Weight Control Breakthrough Of The Century

SIRMANS LOG: 25 NOVEMBER 2014, 1907 HOURS

NEW INJECTION: 24 NOVEMBER 2014, 0853 HOURS

Never in the history of mankind has the poor ever been liberal and moral corrupted until the "New deal" programs created a baby welfare state around 81 years ago. Now we have more poor killing babies in the womb and neutralizing their seed in other ways than any demographic group. No hardship or struggle breeds liberalism and a weak survival instinct.

Anyone with a strong survival instinct (like me) will instinctly know the unborn must be protected for the long term survival of the species. The fact is the USA simply cannot and will not survive unless the cruel evil 1938 socialist minimum wage law is repealed. Any and all types of wage or price controls must be removed entirely.

That will set the all powerful free market place free to save the USA and western civilization, too. Look at the immigration problem in the USA and around the world, its going to engulf us, there is no human solution.

However, if the USA free market was set free by repealing the evil 1938 socialist minimum wage law, then a genuine true free market place armed with nature's supreme law of natural selection would solve the problem and save the USA and western civilization, too.

SIRMANS LOG: 24 NOVEMBER 2014, 0853 HOURS

PS: I believe they are really fixing to financially knife and gut our beloved military like never before.

WE AFRICAN AMERICANS ARE NOW TREATED LIKE A BUCK TOOTH REDHEADED STEP CHILD BY THE DEMS

Political speaking African Americans are now the

redheaded step child of the Democrat party. This child
has a dependency slave mentality and is totally loyal to
his/her care taker. Yet, this child's dependency and
loyalty is taken for granted. And now a new adoptee is
being favored and groomed ahead of this child, sad,
sad.

This child loves and wants to be just like his care taker
in every way. This dependent child sees the
complexion of his care taker and feels that represents
the ideal way one need to be.

However, when the child looks in the mirror he doesn't
look like his care taker physically but mentally wants
to be as much like his care taker as possible. Plus, this
dependent child sees others that look like him as
competitors, or even the enemy in winning the most
favorite one's role by his care taker. That is why
African Americans won't readily support each other in
businesses or otherwise if there is a choice. And the
beat continues on, as long as this child retains his
slave dependency mentality he will not escape his
predicament, ever.

The only way out and for this child to acquire free
objective independent thinking is to shed his
dependent slave mentality. That is a lot easier said
than done. It is much easier to follow the herd than to
veer off into the unknown and entirely fend for
yourself. Also, to take that giant step it is almost
impossible when there is a welfare state promising to
take care of all in need from cradle to grave.

To take the course of least resistance is embedded in
us all. The only thing that is going to get African
Americans to be free thinker and independent minded
is for the crutch to be kicked from under us. To hell
with the victimized mentality, its time African
Americans take responsibility individually and as a race
and feel responsible for their own survival.

Possibly The Greatest Weight Control Breakthrough Of
The Century

Its time we pull up our pants and face down bad behavior, we know right from wrong, enough of this kindergarten blame, blame, blame game. This cancer crime is out of control in our race and we act like its someone else's problem. There was a time when we blacks had self-respect and behaved as well as any race of people. Why should the Dems treat us with respect, they will continually throwing us a bone every now and then and keep treating us like a buck tooth redheaded step child.

If not for this sinister welfare state African Americans would have long ago shed our dependency slave mentality and still have mostly two parent families.
SIRMANS LOG: 22 NOVEMBER 2014, 1406 HOURS

GREAT WRITER FREDDIE L SIRMANS SR GIVES THE ROCK-HARD COLD-STEEL TRUTH ON DOMESTIC ABUSE
All I hear is abuse, abuse, wife abuse, child abuse, women abuse and on and on to no end. Liberal women are almost up in arms; and if it was left up to them they would de-nut all men and make sissies out of all of us. To me there is no mystery here, men are just being men, and it is just cause and effect in action in my view. Men are aggressive creatures by nature and are only doing what they are allowed to get away with. And it is a pipe dream to expect law enforcement to do more than put a dent in it.

It takes fighting fire with fire to really stamp out or completely get under control domestic type violence of this sort. It takes a lot of loved ones that are willing to make a personal sacrifice to truly stamp out or control domestic violence. There has always been some domestic abuse but never out of control like what we are seeing today.

Possibly The Greatest Weight Control Breakthrough Of The Century

What we are seeing today is the result of a lack of the strong nuclear and extended family unit. Today we have too few no-none-sense kick-ass dads or brothers that are prepared to go to hell or prison before they will tolerate this sort of abuse on a love one. We are too busy using the "N" word on each other to give a damn. Very few cousins or good friends are prepared to make such a sacrifice.

I have personally heard a few men say that the only thing keeping me off her ass is her dad would kill me. Sure, law enforcement will do their job and enforce the law, but no law enforcement agency can protect private citizens 24-7 day in and day out. Even if women are the weaker sex old man colt solved that imbalance many, many years ago by creating an equalizer. But, the thing about that is not all of us have the will or the guts to send a S.O.B. to hell. SIRMANS LOG: 19 SEPTEMBER 2014, 2216 HOURS

It really is a waste of time trying to get a liberal to understand freedom and a free market place. That is why most of the world is poor and will always be poor. The point I'm making is liberals don't really understand freedom. Freedom means every individual has a free choice. Jobs don't just drop out of heaven, someone just like you and I must create or provide a job.

This is the land of the free and no one puts a gun to anyone's head and forces them to work for minimum wages. Everyone in this great country has the right to create his/her own job or quit any job one doesn't like. Most liberals think it is wrong for some people to enjoy the rich life while most stay poor. Right now if the liberals had the power they would take almost everything from the rich and spend it on social programs.

They are too shallow minded to realize that rich people are not stupid. They really believe rich people would

17

continue producing and providing jobs while almost all
of their earnings are being taken away. I just can't
understand how anyone with any common sense could
be so shallow, but they are, and are running the
country, too.

There never has and never will be a rich and wealthy
nation without a lot of rich greedy people to make it
happen. If left entirely up to the liberals the USA would
in no time be a third world nation. Yet, enough wanting
something for nothing voters keep the tax and spend
liberals in power while the country goes to hell in a
hand basket.

SIRMANS LOG: 12 JANUARY 2014, 2341 HOURS

**A HALF OF A LOAF IS BETTER THAN NOTHING!
IF YOU THINK IT'S GETTING BAD NOW WITH
OBAMACARE, YOU HAVEN'T SEEN NOTHING YET,
YOU JUST WAIT, IF THE DEM'S WIN ANYTHING
IN NOV. 2014, THEN WE WILL GET THE FULL
THROBBING PURPLE SHAFT FROM THE
DEMOCRATS. THEY WANT TO FIRST SECURE THE
2014 MIDTERM ELECTION BEFORE THEY RAM
THE FULL SHAFT TO US. IT WILL BE EVEN LESS
JOBS AND A TRILLION MORE IN DEBT. IT WILL
BE LIKE DETROIT CITY NATIONWIDE! THINK
ABOUT IT, WE WILL THEN GET ALL OF
OBAMACARE, AND DRY, TOO. GOD, I ASK IN
YOUR NAME SAVE THIS GREAT NATION.**

It doesn't bother me a lot when I don't sell a lot of
books. That is because I estimate only around 2
percent of the American population has the depth and
wisdom to truly understand what the hell I be talking
about. So be it, I carry on.

They can't get pass the fact that it is not the amount of
money that truly matters; it is the buying power that
really counts. Before the New deal which started the

welfare state $5.00 would buy more than $50.00 will today.

Repealing the minimum wage law would put the provider role back into the hands of the people and allow this great country to survive. Otherwise, there is no way in hell the USA is going to survive on its present course.

Just keep on believing in this phony minimum wage economy and without a doubt within a year I will be proven right. We'll soon see just how nutty my predictions are.

The repeal of the minimum wage law is our savior, but, 98 percent of the population can't get pass believing more and bigger is always better. But, to me a half of a loaf is better than nothing because nothing is what this nation is going to get if we don't change course.
SIRMANS LOG: 29 DECEMBER 2013, 1022 HOURS

MAN/WOMAN OVERBOARD, USA ECONOMY SHIP IS BEGINNING TO SINK!
Folks, I'm just a lowly unknown writer out here pounding away trying to get through to thick sculls. Very few actually know about me or my books, and most of those that do are not interesting in tough accountability and responsibility. But, I know without a doubt at some point my writing will be vindicated.

Reality is reality there is just no way of getting around that fact. Sure, sometimes it takes a while for the results to catch up but there are no free rides in life someone always pays. The liberals and Dem's have been very successful; they have created masses upon masses of government dependents. They have convinced these dependents that government will always be there to take care of them and their needs.

That is not reality that is the biggest lie that has ever been told. There has never been a government that didn't go broke at some point. The free market place made the USA the most richest and powerful nation to ever exist. The government didn't do that, the free market place did that. Now, I believe most of the people running our government today doesn't even believe in a free market place.

I believe most of the people in charge of our government today are socialist or communist at heart. Everyone seems to be so surprised about how the liberals and Dem's connived and forced Obamacare down our throats. There is nothing new here about liberals in my view. How in the hell do you think the liberals and Dem's held on to the USA house of Representative for 40 consecutive years.

They did it by lying and conniving, and that is what is really happening with this Obamacare website. They will never let it work right before the November 2014 election. They intend to keep the confusion going and never let all of the high costs be widely known before the 2014 election. But, God help us if the Dem's win anything in November 2014, because if they do they are going to ram the full purple shaft to this free nation, e.g. Obamacare dry like it or not.

I believe these people are hardcore ideologues and will go down with the ship before yielding an inch, and believe me that is exactly what is about to happen. Trust me, this USA economy ship is taking on too big of a load and is beginning to sink. This ship is going down unless most of its government load is jettisoned, and fast.

However, the only way to lighten governments load is to kick it out of its social and family provider role. And the way to do that is repeal the minimum wage law or else, this economy ship is going down. I suspect many

of the rats have already left the ship in spirit and have
property in in places like New Zealand and Australia.
SIRMANS LOG: 26 DECEMBER 2013, 1840 HOURS

WHO IS THE AFRICAN AMERICAN COMMUNITY'S DADDY?

I'm fixing to briefly weigh in on something I have no
business touching, besides, some people think of me
as a nut case anyway. What if I am off the beaten path
that don't mean my beliefs are wrong. Even a broken
clock is right twice a day. Concerning two great black
athletes that is at loggerheads: Long before O. J. got
into trouble, guess who was always on his case for
being too white? Go figure? Some people just naturally
goes against the grain, enough said. The problem with
the African American race as a whole is culture.

The welfare state has destroyed the African American
family structure and community. But, that don't mean
we have to take it lying down and still not feel
responsible for our own behavior and survival. I don't
have the power to stop anything, but you can bet your
bottom dollar that I will never make excuses for bad
behavior. And no matter who does it I'm not accepting
any excuses because of what happened in the distance
past.

Grow up African Americans and take responsibility for
the behavior of yourself and that of your race. This
welfare state has destroyed accountability and
responsibility throughout all of America and I'm sick
and tired of it. Today a decent law abiding black man
can't walk into many stores without being feared
because we as a race won't clean up our own
community house.

Don't tell me that ain't from a lack of feeling
responsible for our own behavior as individuals and as
a race. We still have a dependent slave mentality and

21

think it's the white mans fault. The only cure for that is for someone to kick the crutch from under us and demand we stand on our own two feet. Independent minded people don't look to blame and find excuses to fail. I know I may sounds cold, but this USA economy is fixing to collapse and we black folks need to wake up and be prepared, now.

Every preacher in the pulpit and any member in the black community with an ounce of authority need to feel responsible for this cancer in our community called crime. I don't mean taking any physical action we have law enforcement for that. What I'm talking about is taking a moral stand instead of not feeling racially responsible for bad behavior in our youth.

If we don't save our youths no other race will. I didn't intend to vent like this, I just got carried away but something's need to be said. The so called African American leadership is out to lunch.

SIRMANS LOG: 18 DECEMBER 2013, 1750 HOURS

THERE IS NO GOVERNMENT SYSTEM EVER TO EXIST MORE SELF-DESTRUCTIVE THAN A WELFARE STATE!

Like a junkie on the streets trying to get a fix there is nothing a welfare state won't sell off to support its seized social and family provider role. As long as the USA government stays in its social and family provider role it will be impossible for the USA to stop reckless spending or survive.

Right now, the liberals doesn't have the survival instinct or the wisdom to see a real need to stop spending. They are living in the moment and can't see any real danger in reckless spending, and you couple that with an economically ignorant main stream press and general public, all I know to do is pray.

Possibly The Greatest Weight Control Breakthrough Of The Century

Abolishing the minimum wage law will give the social and family provider role back to the people where it belongs and has always been until the "New deal" seized it in 1938. God I ask in your name, "Save the USA." Time is a winding down, I don't know how much we have left, but, I know beyond a shadow of doubt that a total economic collapse is near unless drastic changes are made.

When I look at the future I think the republicans will soon get the power to have their shot at this health care thing. But, I have news for them too, just like the Dem's they think government can keep and hold on to its social and family provider role, wrong.

I believe unless the republicans and conservatives set about abolishing the minimum wage law they will be seen as phony liberals and quickly replaced. But, of course do like the Dem's never admit in advance what your real intentions are, just git in there and rid the country of this Minimum wage law. It's a free market place killer. See Sirmans survival plan further down.

Most of the big cities water, sewage, and bridges infrastructure were built before a minimum wage law, so, don't tell me junking the minimum wage law won't save this great nation. And here is the real kicker: The USA economy is still the economic engine of the world and if it collapses it takes the world economy down with it. Sure, the world economy may bail us, but not before owning us.

The apple cart has been upset and the only thing that can save the USA is a true free market place. Pure communism and socialism never has and never will work, but, now we have a new monster far worse than both of those systems to contend with, it's called the welfare state. There is no system ever to exist more self-destructive than a welfare state.

Possibly The Greatest Weight Control Breakthrough Of The Century

It leaves almost no survival tools in place to survival on when nature's bust cycle comes around or if the economy collapses. It really is no joke when I say it may be all the way back to the Stone age for modern civilization. We have no strong nuclear and extended family system to survive on. We have centralized factory farming for our meats and vegetables and hardly any small farmers and home gardeners.

That means we have no adequate emergency backup bartering capacity if the economy collapses and money is worthless. And on and on, our family morals and values would make dog eat dog look like a Sunday picnic after a week into a collapse. Wages and prices must be free floating for a genuine free market place to work and that can't happen with a minimum wage law or any kind of wage or price control.

The consumer cost of living is what's going to kill off the USA economy and Obamacare just speeds up the process. Here is the Ultimatum: Either the USA government abolish the minimum wage law which will free the people to save themselves and the country, or it tries to consolidate and hold on to its current social and family provider role.

If it chooses the latter there is no doubt in my mind that it will to no avail sell off the country to foreigners to try to hang on to a role it shouldn't be in, in the first place. You just watch, and the wait won't be very long. I can dissect an economy as well as anyone and that is what I predict is going to happen. You can't get blood out of a turnip.

I doubt there is any gold left at Fort Knox and there is no telling what else has already been sold off by the federal reserve. I'm telling you as a man of great super natural wisdom, unless the minimum wage law is abolished we might as well kiss our freedom and this great country good by forever.

Possibly The Greatest Weight Control Breakthrough Of The Century

SIRMANS LOG: 04 DECEMBER 2013, 2217 HOURS

AMERICA! YOU HAVE BEEN SOLD A FALSE BILL OF GOODS

There is a sucker born everyday. It amazes me how gullible people are. They have fallen for this cock & bull big lie that the Obamacare website is somehow a big screw-up, wrong. I for one don't buy that for one second. A computer or a website must obey what it is programmed to do.

The problem is: There is no way in the hell liberals and Dem's are going to let it be known on a large scale the double and triple cost the people will face until after November 2014. Get a grip America; you have been sold a false bill of goods. And be prepared for a never ending list of excuses, but, you will never get a proper working website with cost no matter what you are told. I rest my case.

SIRMANS LOG: 30 NOVEMBER 2013, 2216 HOURS

FINAL SOLUTION TO THE RACE AND ECONOMIC PROBLEM IN THE USA AS SEEN BY GREAT WRITER FREDDIE L SIRMANS SR., A MUST READ.

UPDATED VERSION: AFRICAN AMERICAN EXCUSES, EXCUSES, EXCUSES, AND I'M SICK AND TIRED OF IT. WRITER ATTACKS BLACK LEADERSHIP.

Halt, stop, or brace yourself, because this great writer is fixing to let her rip, go on a tirade, rant, or what ever you may call it. OK, lets just dispense with any bull s... and just talk plain turkey. Sure, there is a lot of racism in America, always has been and always will be. Hell, I may be called a racist, but I think not.

Possibly The Greatest Weight Control Breakthrough Of
The Century

Life is not perfect and this nation is not perfect, but it
is the greatest country to ever exist in my view. I love
this great country and it is the only home that I have
ever known. This great country offers the most
individual freedom and opportunity to ever exist on
earth, and it still does in spite of our beloved tax and
spends liberals, but still I love-um like a brother.

Now, as to my beloved African American race, the
problem with us is too much pampering, period. Hell,
I'm a neurotic mentally handicapped cripple from my
childhood bed wetting days, yet I will never stoop to
being just a plain excuse maker. If one accepts
excuses for failure an excuse can always be found.

Sure, there may be be a good reason for an excuse,
but as for my self I don't want to hear it, I only accept
results. Like a coach once said: "you show me a good
loser, and I'll show you a loser." I have been counted
out all of my life. For me, I have always taken
responsibility for my own survival and I know beyond a
shadow of doubt that otherwise I wouldn't be standing
today.

Today all I hear from African American leadership is
what we lack, what we don't have, we don't have jobs,
and on and on. However, the question that needs to be
asked is: What do we need to do for our community
our selves? Duh! And they will all look at each other
like helpless sheep. Number one should be how could
we provide more of our own jobs in our communities.

Possibly The Greatest Weight Control Breakthrough Of
The Century

We African Americans have our racial priorities mixed
up or maybe even misplaced in my view. Everyone's
priority should be immediately family first, then
community, city, state, country, but ones race can
never be totally ignored to fit somewhere in that
order.

One must have a mental identity to know who he/she
really is as a person; otherwise one could end up with
no true racial identity. Something of the sort has
happened to the African American race on a mass
scale.

We African Americans as a race mentally see ourselves
as dependent like siblings that can't do for ourselves
and must be taken care of by the master. And like
most siblings we are jealous and compete against each
other for the master's favors. That is why you see the
herd mentality and we always vote anywhere from 90
percent to 99 percent for one party in almost every
election.

We as a race are locked into this dependent sibling
psyche. It is not a bad thing, it kept the African
American race alive in an almost totally hostile
environment right out of slavery. However,
circumstance and the nation has evolved and that type
of psyche is no longer needed for the black race to
survive. Yet, the welfare state won't let blacks escape
its dependent mentality.

The only thing that can break this dependency chain is

Possibly The Greatest Weight Control Breakthrough Of
The Century

for African Americans to be forced to stand on its own
two feet. Folks, I don't have anything to do with
reality, I am only telling things as I see them, you
have the freedom to totally disagree with anything I
write and brand me a fool and idiot, so be it.

The African American race in America is awesome; we
hold many of the most powerful elected offices in this
great nation, from the office of president on down.
There is no logical reason why African Americans can't
employ at least a quarter of the jobs in its own
communities, yet I doubt its over 3 percent.

For God sake, grow up African Americans, grab the bull
by the horns, and learn to love all people and
especially those that look like you. Now, don't you go
telling me you don't have hate and contempt for those
that look like you? Otherwise, why else would there be
all of this mass killings in black communities?

Plus, where you spend your money proves where your
first loyalty priority lies and it's certainly not with the
man in the mirror. No one is expected to support a
dirty greasy spoon eatery, but remember Auburn
Avenue and the likes in other cities could equal the
best before the welfare state came about. Now, our
elites run as far as affordable away from an all black
neighborhood and it is all because of our welfare
state.

The welfare state has reduced the once proud Negro
race to a bunch of government dependent siblings that
are constantly at each others throat. We don't trust

each other or truly respect each other and is ashamed of an all black neighborhood. And don't give me this bull excuse about high crime, the movie "Raising in the sun" proves blacks couldn't wait to get out long before crime was a problem.

If you don't love who you really are how can you expect other races to respect you. Liberalism is responsible for this sad condition and to this day still patronizes African Americans and hates nothing more than a black that wants to be self sufficient and independent. A black conservative threatens liberals ability to keep African Americans dependent minded and self-rejecting more than anything else.

You black man, you don't truly love your own people, you mentally see yourself like your master and better than that sassy nigger that is undeserving of respect. Besides, you see that sassy nigger as a competitor against you, why should you kiss his ass and help him to get ahead, f... him, I'll spend my money where I want too, and anyone that's got a problem with that can kiss my black ass. This is the type of thinking that goes on in the minds of so many in the African American community.

The only thing that can break this locked-in African American dependency mentality is to kick the young eagle out of the welfare state nest, then it will be forced to fly on its own, that is what the mother eagle does. What I just said is not cold and uncaring, that is being prepared to survive on ones own, and not disappear off this earth when this welfare state soon crashes.

The African American sad condition is the tip of the
USA survival spear, or the canary in our culture mine.
God save my beloved homeland. Hallelujah.

OK, OK, having aired it out and said my peace, what is
the real solution to the African American problem?
Anyone familiar with my work should know my
constant drum beat for the only thing that can save all
of America and even western civilization.

It is the economy, fool! Nothing on earth is more
powerful than a genuine true free market place
economy; it trumps the law and everything in terms of
having and maintaining an orderly society.

However, the USA liberal socialist destroyed our true
free market place economy almost eighty years ago by
enacting the evil 1938 socialist minimum wage law.
And the inner fabric of moral decay and culture rot
along with a lack of any emergency bartering capacity
has grown unabated ever since.

A true free market place economy must be absolutely
free to have the power to discipline itself and the
nation, the same as Mother Nature, with its supreme
law of natural selection. There must be a survival need
for anything in nature to exist, otherwise it starts
ceasing to exist based on nature's supreme law of
"Natural selection."

The enacting of the 1938 minimum wage law gave the

Possibly The Greatest Weight Control Breakthrough Of The Century

USA government for the first time absolute power over private property rights and business production and distribution. That act for the first time allowed liberals to seize almost absolute power by operating a candy store and promising the moon and back.

Before the 1938 minimum wage law it was almost impossible to inflate the USA currency because the economy had the discipline power to purge out inflation, waste, inefficiency and the likes. Now, the minimum wage law acts as a purge inhibitor and every imaginable negative anti-survival special interest group in America have grown like wild flowers unabated ever since. Mass killing's in the womb and same sex marriages are just new additions to the anti-survival paths the USA is going down.

Negative anti-survival special interest is now a swamp with the coalition power to take down this great nation. Creating our minimum wage law purge inhibitor is like trying to stop nature's life and death cycle, insane. The evil 1938 socialist minimum wage law have an almost over-powering appeal to the economically ignorant, and has all but destroyed our culture, good morals, and any capacity to barter.

A nation can't have emergency bartering capacity without enough small farmers and home gardeners, which is what got the USA through the great depression. I could go on and on with the destruction this evil 1938 socialist minimum wage law has done to this great nation.

Possibly The Greatest Weight Control Breakthrough Of
The Century

But, I will wrap it up by saying this: Everybody and his brother has an opinion, but it is my God given destiny to let you know until the 1938 minimum wage law is repealed it is impossible for the USA to be saved. The "Final solution" is to repeal this evil law, or we perish, period.

I believe all to no avail the federal reserve and politicians trying to save this welfare state beast will eventually sell the nations sovereignty, land, wealth, and mineral rights off like a hooker on the block. Plus, there is no telling what has already been sold off being $18,000,000,000,000 in debt already.

Only a handful of people know, but I seriously doubt there is any gold left at Fort Knox anymore. I can't make anybody believe me; still I believe I understand the workings of an economy as well as anyone. And I promise you this weak phony P…. of an economy the USA have today is almost as useless as tits on a boar hog in terms of saving itself or this great nation.

Repeal the 1938 minimum wage law and give the USA economy back its original power, please Sir/Madam. It is not about how much increase in wages that really count, it is about having a job to buy enough food and necessities to survive at all. What good is a higher wage if you can't afford hardy anything, duh? It won't happen overnight, but repealing the minimum wage law will wean inflation out of our currency so $1.00 will buy what $20.00 will today.

Folks, I don't have to be right on my assessment, and

I even hope I'm proven wrong. Why oh Lord, why have I been blessed with so much raw wisdom, it is like a curse, I see things so clearly, why me o-lord. Writer answers that himself: Why not you. Amen.
SIRMANS LOG: 07 MAY 2015, 1328 HOURS.

WRITER'S EXPERIENCE:
We all have our demons and fears and sometimes an out of control ego, but one should never forget that nothing can overpower one's will.

If one will just face and look at all things one will discover that facades abounds. Failure to face and stare down ones own demons is why so many tries to escape through alcohol and drugs.

CAN THE REPUBLICAN ESTABLISHMENT STOP THE "DONALD" BEFORE HE CROSSES THE 2016 PRESIDENTIAL FINISHING LINE?
It is my experience with family members and those with severe flaws; they can force one into making a deep hard emotional choice that may defy reason. With some people you have to either love them or leave them there is no shallow middle ground. I believe that is the case with Mr. Trump's supporters, they have made their love choice. Still, it is the issues that nurture this love.

Almost everyone knows love can be blind. Many parents have learned the hard way it is not wise to put down an undesirable suitor. Mr. Trump's supporters know who he is and are not looking for a Mr. perfect. They made their choice and who is to say they are wrong, I can't, only God knows. Just like in a marriage, the ones almost everyone predicts will fail, often don't, and vice-versa.

No matter what anyone may think Mr. Trump has a great issue focused formula for winning. But, I feel there is a diplomatic character element that makes the formula seems more of a vice than a virtue to the majority.

Take away the stinging insults, the cold harsh put downs, and the eye for eye that leaves everyone blind, and then you have a pure non-stoppable winner in my view. There is no doubt he has the issues the Republican Party has totally ignored.

There is no secret here, anyone could take these same issues and get the same results Mr. Trump is getting, but a cold harsh voice of authority is a must or you won't be believed or trusted.

However, I may be totally wrong on this whole matter, Mr. Trump may still rule the roost, who really knows? "No chain is stronger than its weakest link".

Free speech and the truth shall set you free. But, liberalism and ignorance doesn't want to hear the truth unless it agrees with it. The first and second amendments to the US. constitution must prevail at all cost, lets don't get it twisted, y'all.

I thank God for any man/woman that won't lie down and rollover, and is willing to stand up for all of our first amendment rights. Praise be to God.

It is now the welfare state or we; so, starving the welfare beast out of existence is the only way of getting back to sanity before we all are over-run and praying five times a day.

Anyone that thinks that the USA or any welfare state

can be saved without first getting rid of its minimum wage law is a fool in my view. Sure, I may be the one that is really the fool, but I'm sure history will prove me right on this.

I wrote on my website FLSirmans.com a while back that Mr. Trump was just the catalyst before the main event that is going to save this great country. As a super great writer of almost supernatural wisdom I still stand by my first observation. However, only God knows how or when the main event will take the stage. Who knows?

Right now currency-wise all of the USA survival eggs are in one basket, which is a sad dangerous situation. The value of the coin portion of the USA currency must be return back to being within itself, such as real gold, real silver, real copper, or some other precious medal, period.

Otherwise, when this world economy soon collapses the USA will be back to trade and bartering to survive, but with very, very few small farmers and home gardeners almost no one will have anything to eat or barter with, dooms day will be upon us.

No western civilization problems such as immigration, crime, morals, economics etc. today will ever be controlled without first getting rid of all minimum wage laws. The reason is simple: The core or main problem with the west today is self-destruction; it lacks self-societal discipline, due to the minimum wage laws.

In a free society only the economy can maintain proper societal discipline in the long run contrary to the law as almost everyone thinks. Plus, minimum wage laws chokes off the purging power of a true free market place economy and leaves it with no power to maintain societal discipline.

Possibly The Greatest Weight Control Breakthrough Of
The Century

Today, with hardly any societal discipline left there is very little means of stopping liberalism and ignorance from bringing on our total self-destruction. Far too many people today believe survival is owed to them and it is always someone else's fault if they fail. Liberalism and ignorance has no true concept of what it takes for this great USA nation to survive, financial or otherwise, period.
SIRMANS LOG: 08 MARCH 2016, 2018 HOURS.

WHY SOME PEOPLE SEEM TO BE LOVED AND ACCEPTED NO MATTER WHAT THEY DO OR SAY
There is an old axiom that has befuddled reasonable men and women forever. It is the saying that "To those whom much is given, much is expected". Hell, I feel it may even be a law of nature.

I believe people tend to love and accept you the way you truly are to yourself. And if you are truly a talented and responsible person that is the way people expect you to act. I think that is why liberals can get away with far more than a no nonsense responsible conservative can, the expectation is not the same.

I think that is why anyone with great and proper character that goes down and wallow in the gutter is not living up to his/her expectation, period, and will be treated accordingly. It may not be fair but that is just the way it is.

Some people the more they act up and act a fool are written off with low expectation and just loved anyway in spite of their behavior. We all have at least one those in the family. My grand mother used to always say, "It takes all kind to make up a world".

In many families one or two people always complain, why am I always expected to carry more than my

share of the load. Tough titty, that is just the way it is.
Never forget, nature is all about maintaining a balance
in the universe.

When you see an extreme it is only creating a
counterbalance against another extreme somewhere.
Remember what Nixon said about one of his tough
guys, sure, he is a S.O.B. but he is our S.O.B.
SIRMANS LOG: 05 MARCH 2016, 1045 HOURS.

A QUICK WORLD ECONOMY FACT:
No matter what the world economic condition may
seem, the USA is still by far the economic engine for
the world. The big Dragons, the little Dragons, and all
others would in no time be in the poor house if the
USA economy heart skips a few beats. There is no
other market that even comes close to the size of the
USA market.
SIRMANS LOG: 12 MARCH 2016, 1614 HOURS.

USA LEADERS FIDDLE WHILE ROME BURNS.
KNOWLEDGE IS POWER BABY:
As a writer of almost supernatural wisdom I offer a
USA survival blueprint why not follow it. If a better one
exists, please disregard. Sure, You can laugh, but
history will be the final judge. You have been
enlightened, you know the one and only thing that
must be done, now get it done.

Me, this little lone neurotic writer attacking this big
giant liberalism Ogre is like David attacking Goliath.
Don't look a gift horse in the mouth.

NOTICE:
 I will almost always say bridle liberalism. The reason
is liberalism is not necessarily a bad thing in fact
liberalism makes a more caring and better world, but it
will also destroy everything if not disciplined and kept

under control. Either an iron fist literally type government or a government with a true free market place economy can keep liberalism bridled.

Since 1938 the USA no longer has a true free market place economy due to the government enforced minimum wage law. And without a true free market place economy the USA has no way to maintain societal discipline thereby allowing liberalism to take down this great nation.

These do-good make everything right liberals are on a warpath about gun control, they can barely sit still and are wiggling in their seats. What they don't understand and are too shallow to realize is out of control liberalism is the cause of the gun problem in the first place.

However, I'm one that believes liberals forcing threatening gun control down the nations throat is the one thing that will definitely give republicans a Trifecta or complete a Hat Trick in 2016.

If you want a better society you first must have a better class of people, period. From lack of societal discipline this USA nation is being over run with moral decay and culture rot, that is where the real problem lies. Almost all of this nations old tried and true norms and traditions have been corrupted by liberalism.

They have been replaced by new insane anti-survival norms like same sex marriages and mass killing of future unborn babies in the womb. I won't preach, I will end by saying you have been enlightened on what must be done to save the USA from total doom.

Gun violence is one of the least of this nation's problems, our way of life and survival itself is on a slow countdown. And here we are fiddling while Rome burns.

Possibly The Greatest Weight Control Breakthrough Of The Century

As a writer of almost supernatural wisdom I have said a thousand times the one sure thing that will save the USA from total doom, so there is no excuse why this great nation should go the way of the great Auk (Click on >) Auk.

No matter which way the wind blows, I'm here to warn you that only a genuine true free market economy with no kind of government wage or price control can provide the discipline to save the USA and western civilization, period.

You see, only an economy without any kind of government wage or price control will have the necessary purging power not only to discipline and protect itself, but will also protect the nation's culture, moral, and spiritual values from over powering rot and decay like what is eating us alive today.

Repeal the insane arch-evil 1938 socialist minimum law now. Let the only thing that can possibly save the USA and western civilization, which is a genuine true free market place economy with no choking government wage or price controls, what so ever work its miracle.

Agree or not, like it or not, without a doubt I am right on this, I will bet the farm on it. There are certain things about human nature that never changes, things such as spite, envy, jealousy, hate, superstition, and the rest of our emotions. Things of this sort haven't changed one iota in over 2000 years.

Concerning societal discipline: As late as the nineteen fifties or sixties many small towns and rural areas in the USA didn't even bother to lock their doors. So, concerning societal discipline what has changed in today's world, the key word is discipline. The USA has practical no societal discipline left today.

Possibly The Greatest Weight Control Breakthrough Of
The Century

That is the main reason we have so many nuts
committing mass killings with guns today. It takes
discipline to isolate or weed out those that won't
conform. Sport teams use tryouts to see who conforms
and the military uses basic training to see who
conforms. Well, a healthy society on a much larger
scale must have some means to isolate those unwilling
to conform.

I believe those that has the mentality to go out in a
blaze of hate and terror will always show some tell tale
signs well in advance, its just that those that knows
are not telling or speaking up. Many first grade school
teachers to a high degree can point out even then the
ones most likely to be in trouble with the law eighteen
years later.

I will bet my bottom dollar that at least one person
knew everyone of these mass killers was a danger to
society in some way before they acted. The reason the
USA doesn't have the societal discipline to isolate and
deal with these type of individuals is because of our
minimum wage law. Don't roll your eyes and laugh,
because I know you think that is stupid and doesn't
make sense.

Let me explain, the shallow minded see the minimum
wage law only in terms of how much more money one
is paid on a job and they can't get pass that. Sure,
only a fool wouldn't like to make a living wage or make
more money. And getting any kind of a private sector
pay raise is a good thing and will work. But, on a large
or national scale with everyone getting a forced
government raise it may give everyone more money,
but more purchasing power will be just an illusion.

It is an illusion because every forced government wage
increase results in a higher cost of living increase. And
over time the cost of living increases will far out

Possibly The Greatest Weight Control Breakthrough Of
The Century

distance any salary increases. The minimum wage law
is why twenty years ago ones salary versus cost-of-
living would buy far more in the grocery store then
than it will today. And if moral decay and culture rot
doesn't doom the USA first consumer cost of living
soon will.

Buying power is what truly and really counts, not more
and more lesser and lesser-valued inflated dollars,
which the shallow minded and less informed can't
seem to comprehend.

Yet, if the government raised the minimum wage ten
dollars it would kill off most small businesses and
consumer-cost-of-living would really sky rocket even
more. Anyone that know the basics of true economics
should know that any kind of government wage or
price control doesn't work in the long run and will rip
apart a nation's culture and moral inner fabric.

The real danger and destruction from any kind of
government imposed wage or price control is what it
does to the entire USA economy. Any kind of
government imposed wage or price control de-nuts
and renders a free market place economy practically
helpless with almost no purging power left. Purging
power is what gives an economy the discipline to
protect itself, the nations culture, moral, and spiritual
values.

Starting in 1938 the USA economy's hands has been
tied behind its back due to the enacting of our
minimum wage law, and ever since then the USA as a
nation has been without societal discipline leaving the
nation almost without a rudder.

Another big problem with the USA economy is the USA
government is trying to manage and control it. That in
itself is an impossible task simply because there is just
too many variables. The government shouldn't be

41

forcing a minimum wage on the private sector and it shouldn't be in the stock market either.

Plus, the biggest no, no of all is for government to ever become a social and family provider. Once that happens there is no peaceful way out for government, because when money starts running out the mobs is going to be coming after politicians with pitchforks. Only repealing the insane arch-evil 1938 socialist minimum wage law can prevent this from happening, otherwise there is not enough societal discipline left to keep western civilization from regressing all the way back to the stone age.

Government should run the country, the military and stick to collecting taxes and get the hell out of the way to allow a genuine true free market place economy to prevail. Government should stay with what it does best collecting taxes, running the country, the military, and leave the economy to the private sector, period.

Plus, that was mainly the way it was before government decided to take over private enterprise by not allowing the private sector to set its own wages and prices (The insane arch-evil 1938 socialist minimum wage law ended private control of the USA economy). And until control of the USA economy is back in the hands of the private sector it is impossible for this nation to survive, period.

As a writer with awesome creative thinking ability along with almost supernatural wisdom I believe even if the republicans do complete a hat trick in 2016 liberalism will still rule the day. In the USA and other welfare states around the world liberalism is on autopilot.

Which means the only thing that can bridle liberalism enough to save western civilization from total doom is a true genuine free market place economy, period.

42

Possibly The Greatest Weight Control Breakthrough Of
The Century

But, here is the catch; it is impossible to have a true genuine free market place economy with any kind of government enforced wage or price control in effect, period.

So, even if the republicans do get a Trifecta in 2016 by gaining control of both houses of congress and the presidency it won't save the USA from total doom, unless the arch-evil 1938 socialist minimum wage law is repealed once and for all.

The only true benefit I can see for a minimum wage law in the first place was to inflate our currency to finance and keep our liberal created welfare state in power. Without a minimum wage law a pure free market place economy will purge out inflation. Now, to change gears, Just like the life and death cycle is necessary for life to exist, the boom and bust cycle in an economy is necessary for an economy to exist. It is a law of nature.

The USA economy is going to collapse that is a given, no one knows when, but a big bust cycle is long overdue. My grave concern is what is going to happen afterward. I'm not out to scare anyone one, I'm just a lone writer with a one man's opinion, and hopefully I'm wrong.

It is just simply impossible for any society to get through a long overdue bust cycle without a strong nuclear and extended family system in place, which the USA no longer has.

Repealing the arch-evil 1938 socialist minimum wage law will restore our strong nuclear and extended family system along with strong morals and spirituals values providing time don't run out on us. Otherwise I can't see any way around total doom, period. You can call me crazy, a nut, or whatever, but that is the way I see it, sorry.

Possibly The Greatest Weight Control Breakthrough Of The Century

Before 1938 a lone woman with a purse could walk through a black neighborhood or any neighborhood at midnight and no one would harm her. Today what has changed, the come about of the insane arch-evil 1938 socialist minimum wage law put a stop to societal discipline. And since that day our once real true free market place economy lacks the purging power to stop inflation, culture rot, or moral decay.

Lets face it, liberalism and its created welfare state has destroyed individual responsibility and accountability to the point that the USA may no longer have the capacity to remain a free people. In spite of out of control liberalism and its created welfare state we in the USA still has the most individual freedom found anywhere in the world.

Only the second amendment is keeping us free, but history is not on us gun owner's side. The insane arch-evil 1938 socialist minimum wage law must be repealed now, not tomorrow. Otherwise, one way or another big stud liberalism is going to eventually have its way with the 2nd amendment in my view.

NOTE:
The worst mistake any conservative with strong great character can commit is try to win the approval of liberalism, because if they can make you a perfectionist then you destroy yourself by dehumanizing yourself.

People don't love you because you are perfect; people love you because you are human. Never constantly deny any negative, make one statement per negative, then repeat that has been addressed and move on, period.

Remember, rightly or wrongly no one likes a whiner.

44

Possibly The Greatest Weight Control Breakthrough Of The Century

Let them take a hike if they can't take a joke.
SIRMANS LOG: 06 NOVEMBER 2015, 0018 HOURS.

GREAT WISDOM:
Lately I'm hearing a constant drum beat from conservatives and republicans on cutting taxes to save the USA from doom. Sorry, it is too late for that liberalism is much too embedded and powerful and will come roaring back with a vengeance if this path continues.

I agree under normal circumstance that should be the normal thing to do, but the masses upon masses of government dependents at the first sign of real pain politically is going to send conservatives and republicans packing.

The better and only way, again I repeat if conservatives and republicans have any chance of saving the USA from doom they must repeal the insane arch-evil 1938 socialist minimum wage law, then a true genuine free market place economy will kick in and do whatever it takes to save this great nation.

It is a one shot chance, if it is not taken or misses the mark, shallow minded liberalism will once and for all drive the final nail into our coffin, this I guarantee.

Only a true free market place economy has the power to bridle liberalism enough to have a fighting chance of saving the USA from total doom, period.
SIRMANS LOG: 29 OCTOBER 2015, 1754 HOURS.

BRIEF FOOD FOR THOUGHT ADD ON:
Sure, the rich and powerful has always aborted and killed babies in and out of the womb. But, as to the

rest of society mass killing of future unborn babies in the womb is a modern thing within the last fifty years no matter the reason.

Nothing has advanced civilization more than conquering armies and in the distance past mass raping almost always was seen as just part of the reward bounty. Hell, even in slavery if every life that resulted from rape were aborted there would be a lot fewer blacks around today.

Yet, some blacks are setting on their high horses demanding that every life resulting from a rape be killed in the womb. Studies have shown that the trauma of being a raped victim in many cases is eased by the love from the innocent child. I'm not condoning anything, I'm just saying...

SIRMANS LOG: 27 OCTOBER 2015, 1938 HOURS.

THE POWER OF FORGIVENESS:
What my harshest critics will never understand is no one acquires almost supernatural wisdom without enduring unusual great suffering to survive in some way, period. I feel if I weren't spiritual to the core I would have long fallen by the way side.

It is virtually impossible to mentally destroy anyone that can genuine love and forgive. I just repeat to myself as much as necessary, I can wish all people goodwill through God who strengthens me.

THE ARCH-EVIL DESTRUCTIVE POWER OF A MINIMUM WAGE LAW
If I had to choose just one thing that has all but totally destroyed western civilization and will soon finish it off: That one thing is a government forced minimum wage law on private enterprise.

Possibly The Greatest Weight Control Breakthrough Of The Century

Without a government forced minimum wage law consumer inflation cannot exist to propel a welfare state. It is the welfare state that has produced all of these masses upon masses of dense shallow minded liberal thinkers with no true concept of moral or economic survival, period.

Sure, they think I'm a fool, a hater, or some kind of monster that don't know what the hell I'm talking about. But, I know I'm right on this and we'll all soon find out when this phony USA economy totally collapses and send us all back to the Stone age.
SIRMANS LOG: 25 NOVEMBER 2015, 1122 HOURS.

FREE ADVICE ADD ON:
No one asked my advice, but I decided to give a little free advice anyway. There are two main ways to control or motivate people; it is through love or fear. Some believe love is best but fear is more dependable.

At least in the old days the west had sense enough to prop up strongmen and that kept order, but somehow along the way liberalism creep made that a no, no. Now, almost total disorder abounds, because the west to this day still believes one size fits all.

In many cases involving an army or fighting force it must boil down to option odds, meaning ones chances of surviving is equal or greater staying and fighting than running away. Strongmen shoot deserters on sight.
SIRMANS LOG: 15 NOVEMBER 2015, 0855 HOURS.

WORDS OF GREAT WISDOM:

Possibly The Greatest Weight Control Breakthrough Of The Century

What I keep trying to get through thick sculls is we must bring back a genuine true free market place economy, then the phony climate change liberalism cause, the debt problem, the immigration problem, the health care problem, the crime problem, and every other grave problem we have will solve itself.

Only a true free market place economy has the power to keep liberalism at bay, anything less is like pissing on a barn fire expecting to put it out. These politicians will be making promises until doomsday, yet higher taxes and more debt grows daily.

SIRMANS LOG: 09 NOVEMBER 2015, 1300 HOURS.

FOOTBALL PLAYERS DEMAND:
The purpose for going to school is supposes to be to get an education, period. How long can the USA remain a free people, duh? This is just another sad escalation of liberalism flexing its muscles; get use to it, much more to come.

With a problem of this sort in the final analysis it all boils down to a lack of societal discipline in some way. But, what can you expect, unless our insane arch-evil 1938 socialist minimum wage law is repealed it is impossible for the USA to be saved. We are now entering the early stage where only an iron fist literally can maintain order.

You can't keep individual freedom without self-responsibility, self-accountability, and self-restraint, period. Soon the people will demand that government take away our individual freedoms just to maintain order. Just keep living, you'll see. Liberalism is out of control and deadly.

There is no doubt in my mind that out of control liberalism is going to take the great USA down unless

Possibly The Greatest Weight Control Breakthrough Of
The Century

we get back to a genuine true free market place
economy and soon. I wish I could break my pen and
walk away from this, but it is a calling and I just can't.
**SIRMANS LOG: 08 NOVEMBER 2015, 0045
HOURS.**

BRIEF INSERT:
Like the gospel without exception I'm one that totally
believes in the strong nuclear and extended family
system and the free enterprise system. That gives over
6000 years of proven tried and true survival
experience backing up my writing. So, how can I be a
wrongheaded fool and nut case? Duh?

Welfare states and governments always fail or go
broke sooner or later, only the nuclear and extended
family system and the free enterprise system have
withstood the test of time. The USA nuclear and
extended family system is almost totally destroyed
because there must be a survival "need" for anything
in nature to exist.

The USA government as a social and family provider
welfare state has almost completely eliminated the
survival need for a nuclear and extended family
system, a system that has assured the survival of the
human species for over 6000 years. My God! What a
price the USA is gonna pay for this severe lack of
wisdom. I am talking about the very foundation for
human survival itself.

This could mean back to the Stone Age or even human
extinction. With the awesome almost supernatural
wisdom I have it is a burden to be one of the very few
that can see what's coming our way. No one else has
to believe anything I write. However, I don't write just
to impress anyone, I only write what I truly believe.

Possibly The Greatest Weight Control Breakthrough Of The Century

NOTE:
There is no such thing as a free market place economy with any kind of government enforced wage or price controls, period. However, in the private sector unions should have the power to drive wages as high as they can, but government should stay with collecting taxes and let the free market place police itself.
SIRMANS LOG: 23 DECEMBER 2015, 2050 HOURS.

TRILLION $ USA SPENDING PACKAGE
For the wrong reason in my view the republican establishment is doing the right thing when caving just to hold on to power thereby waiting for a one-punch liberalism knockout. All most of these modern day shallow minded conservatives that can't see the big picture know is to cut here or cut there, which is political suicide when millions upon millions is solely dependent on government for their survival.

Thank God they haven't got their way because the resulting economic pain would definitely have put liberals back in total power and all would be lost maybe forever. As it is the republicans stand a better than fifty fifty chance of getting that one punch liberalism knockout opportunity with a trifecta after November 2016.

Only a one punch knockout blow can bring liberalism under control enough to save the USA and western civilization from total doom. Need I say more, by now most people already knows what my "said" one punch liberalism knockout is? Hint: 1938, Thank God.

I assure you our USA welfare state economy is going to soon totally collapse, it is impossible for it not to. Only by repealing our arch-evil 1938 socialist minimum wage law first can total anarchy back to the stone age be prevented, period.
SIRMANS LOG: 17 DECEMBER 2015, 1650 HOURS.

GREAT WRITER, FREDDIE L. SIRMANS SR. GOES OUT ON A LIMB ADDRESSING TERRORISM HOPING IT WON'T BE SAWED OFF.

The west is in a quandary and can't understand why it is so hated and unappreciated instead of loved by some cultures and religions. It is morals and family, fool! Hell, who with even a feeble survival instinct and any sense of true decency not be against out of control liberalism.

If western government forced minimum wage laws on private enterprise is not soon repealed the west will be overrun morally-wise while standing around hugging their pets. The quickest way to destroy any society is for government to do for the people that will weaken their survival instinct by leaving little or no survival challenge to face.

Liberalism and the welfare state for the most part has destroyed the strong survival instinct and common sense in the USA and only getting rid of the minimum wage laws can untie our economy to save us.

The young and unborn is 100 percent of our future that is why strong culture and morality is a must for future survival. Whereas, liberalism tends to live only for self in the now, me first, I want mine, I want it all, and that scares the hell out of certain cultures and religions.

There is nothing on earth more threatening to future survival than out of control liberalism, period. With the mass use of the "Morning after pill", the mass killing of future unborn babies in the womb, and same sex marriages, how can there be a long term future for western civilization?

Already Western Europe and Japan can't repopulate

Possibly The Greatest Weight Control Breakthrough Of The Century

themselves. Plus, I didn't mention the vast amount of men into porn and all of the women with hidden toys, (Prostitution article). Wake up and get a grip America, western civilization is slipping away, fools.

That should scare the hell out of anyone with a strong normal healthy "Survival instinct". Out of control liberalism will surely bury us all unless wise men and women repeal our insane arch-evil 1938 socialist minimum wage law, period.

SIRMANS LOG: 03 DECEMBER 2015, 1600 HOURS

GREAT WRITER'S VIEW ON THE USA GUN PROBLEM AND MODERN ECONOMIC THINKING: Guns have been plentiful in the land of the USA ever since Plymouth Rock (1620). But, never since has there been a problem with guns until after 1938 for a very simple reason. The reason is norms and morals are what determine a nations character.

1938 is when liberalism got its grip on this nations throat with the enacting of the insane arch-evil 1938 socialist minimum wage law. Ever since that day liberalism and the welfare state has gone about destroying the USA nuclear and extended family system and all good moral and spiritual values in my view.

That has left the USA today as mostly a nation of shallow naive government dependents that see government as some kind of omnipotent sow with nipples that can be sucked on forever.

I pity the fool that thinks the USA economy ship is unsinkable and can take on just one more free load to no end.

Wisdom, wisdom, wisdom, the dumb and stupid thing about depending on a government and welfare state for survival is it destroys the nuclear and extended family system.

There have never been and never will be a society that survived without a strong nuclear and extended family system. In terms of human survival the nuclear and extended family system is everything, and when you destroy that neither the government nor anything else can survive for very long, period.

Repealing the insane arch-evil 1938 socialist minimum wage law will begin restoring the USA only savior the all-powerful "Nuclear and extended family unit". It is not a matter of the USA economy collapsing, it is a matter of how soon.

I've said this before, now I will say it again. Only a genuine true free marketplace economy has the power to save the USA and Western Europe. However, the key is it is impossible to have a genuine true free marketplace economy with any kind of government "Forced" price or wage control law in effect.

There is no greater survival guarantee on earth than a genuine true free marketplace, period.
The biggest mistake in modern economic thinking is the belief that government can manage and control an economy successful over time.

Government managing an economy over time is an impossible task because there are just too many variables. If government would just keep hands off a true free marketplace economy would manage and control itself. A genuine true free marketplace has no favorites and the powers that be always hate that.

Before 1938 government stayed mostly with just collecting taxes and running the country. And let the private sector set its own prices and wages the way it was ever since the founding of the country.

Possibly The Greatest Weight Control Breakthrough Of
The Century

Basically ever since 1938 liberalism and a welfare state
mentality has been running the USA economy. And it is
impossible for this great nation to ever be saved unless
the private sector gets back to setting its own prices
and wages, period.

I am a man of almost supernatural wisdom and can be
wrong on many things, but not on the "Must" for the
private sector being free to set its own prices and
wages if the USA economy is to survival long term, or
at all.

The "Key" to long term economic survival is the
response to market forces, a private sector genuine
true free market place does that well, government
never responds to market forces. That is why unless
drastic basic structure changes are made soon it will
be impossible for the USA economy to survive very
much longer, period. And you can take that to the
bank.

Unless a basic structure change like the private sector
being free to set its own prices and wages again the
USA will soon unravel morally, spiritual, as well as
financially.
SIRMANS LOG: 05 JANUARY 2016, 1908 HOURS.

WHAT IS A PRESIDENTIAL EXECUTIVE ORDER?
One of the biggest misunderstood things in the USA
today is a presidential executive order. A presidential
executive order is suppose to be basically the same as
any CEO or company leader issuing an order to his/her
supervisors, managers, and employees.

Before 1938 a presidential executive order had almost
no effect on the private sector because very few
people depended on government for anything. Today

government is so big with so many agencies that the private sector is almost totally ruled by government.

President Richard Milhouse Nixon is the one that kicked in the door to the imperial presidency, now, our imperial presidency is a well established fact.
SIRMANS LOG: 03 JANUARY 2016, 1214 HOURS.

CURRENT EVENT PASSING THOUGHT?
The predominant shallow minded liberal news media allowed Trump to dominate the news as long as he went mostly after republicans. Now, here comes this down in the gutter Cosby soap opera thing? Come on now? Give me a break, y'all.
SIRMANS LOG: 30 DECEMBER 2015, 1636 HOURS.

WRITER'S BELIEF:
I BELIEVE FORGIVENESS ADVANCES CIVILIZATION AND UN-FORGIVENESS REGRESSES CIVILIZATION. I BELIEVE WITHOUT THE CHRISTIAN RELIGION CIVILIZATION WOULD STILL BE BACK IN THE DARK AGES. THE TRUTH SHALL SET YOU FREE.
SIRMANS LOG: 31 JANUARY 2016, 0059 HOURS.

WHAT IS A LIBERAL OR PROGRESSIVE?
A jurist once said something to this effect, I can't tell you what obscenity is but I know it when I see it. A lot of liberals are claiming that many of our founding fathers were liberals, I say hogwash. Well, I know this, before 1938 and our welfare state about the only place you could find a true liberal was in a rich family or maybe on a college campus for a very simple reason.

Just facing the elements and the day-to-day struggle to stay warm and keep food on the table made just about everyone a conservative or you wouldn't

survive. There was no social or welfare state support
system. And it was almost unheard of for a poor black
woman to kill a future unborn baby in the womb.

Now, today the poor has the worst morals and are
killing more babies in the womb than any other
demographic group, all because no one is instilling
proper norms and traditions in their young. So, how do
you like me now?
SIRMANS LOG: 27 JANUARY 2016, 1615 HOURS.

ESTABLISHED FACTS ADD ON:
Other than an authoritarian type government system,
it is impossible to keep a disciplined orderly society
without a strong nuclear and extended family system
and a genuine true free market place economy. Only
adhering to the above said facts can our liberalism
swamp be drained to saved the USA from total doom.

Politically it really doesn't matter what party wins what
or which individual wins, the USA is past the point of
no return toward total doom. And all is lost unless our
vast liberalism swamp can be drained, period. The only
thing that can save us, hint (1938).

Everything about nature either cycles or ebbs and
flows. That is why a genuine true free market place
economy will automatically protect itself and a nation
through good and bad times. However, liberalism put a
stop to that by enacting the insane arch-evil 1938
socialism minimum wage law to buy votes. And until
that catastrophic mistake is rectified it is impossible for
the USA economy to recover or survive, period.

Sure, the establishment has failed us big time, but,
what is far worse is to go chasing after falling stars at
the end of a rainbow, which I believe is happening. I
say go, follow your star, I hope you find your pot of
gold. I wish you only the best and hope your future will

be bright. As for me: I will continue to count my
blessings and keep the faith, praise be to God.

"There is a sucker born everyday. Everything that
glitters is not gold. Those that live on hope die fasting.
The show must go on. The way to hell is paved with
good intentions. The meek not the weak shall inherit
the earth (paraphrased).

The Lord works in mysterious ways. We now have
millions gullible enough to sell the Brooklyn bridge to,
y'all".
SIRMANS LOG: 22 JANUARY 2016, 1342 HOURS.

PASSING THOUGHT ADD ON:
I don't want to be too clear on this, but, going after
the general could be a signal that justice may go hard
in a parallel direction soon in my view???
SIRMANS LOG: 20 JANUARY 2016, 1253 HOURS.

TRUMP VERSUS CLINTON:
There is an old saying be careful what you hope and
pray for because you just might get it. I believe the
Democratic Party establishment and liberal news media
have in the past and still do believe Senator Clinton
can take Trump in a general election. In other words,
said parties are hoping and praying these two will be in
the final face off showdown.
SIRMANS LOG: 16 JANUARY 2016, 1244 HOURS.

ANOTHER BIG LIBERALISM TAKE DOWN
I'm one that believes it was liberalism that took Cosby
down. I remember it well when he started preaching
responsibility and accountability concerning African
Americans. Immediately afterward the long knives of
the all powerful liberal entertainment industry and
others came out.

Possibly The Greatest Weight Control Breakthrough Of
The Century

I'm not defending anyone I'm just saying this stuff
happen many years ago. This man has given as much
as $20,000,000 to a single black college and given to
many others, he can't be all bad. Why the knifing now
after so many years?

It is all because he made the mistake of sounding too
much like a conservative. And for the liberals that was
his UN-forgivable sin. They will stop at nothing to try
to totally destroy this man in my view.
SIRMANS LOG: 03 FEBRUARY 2016, 1627 HOURS.

FAITH AND TRUST:
I'm one that has total trust in an all powerful genuine
true free market place economy. If the insane Arch-
evil 1938 socialist minimum wage law were repealed
today there would be no drastic overnight changes.
But, one of the greatest powers and forces on earth
would be set free to save the USA at all cost.

It would be a force of nature just like when a body is in
trauma the brain and vital organs take top priority for
blood and oxygen. I'm all about survival, which too few
seem to realize the dire threat we face.

No one man or a group of men can save the USA it is
too late for that. Only a force of nature and a basic
structure change in the USA economy can save us at
this late stage. The insane Arch-evil 1938 socialism
minimum wage law must be repealed now; tomorrow
may be too late, period. I wash my hands of this
matter.

Don't let the Arch-liberals and socialist fool you. They
all deep down believes power come out of the barrel of
a gun. And knows it is only the gun that is keeping
them from grabbing total power. Thank God for our
2nd amendment. Plus, attacking the rich is always

their first step for a take over because they know the rich is the lifeblood of every free nation.

There never has been and never will be a rich and prosperous nation without a lot greedy rich people with a sense of altruism to make it happen, period.

SIRMANS LOG: 06 FEBRUARY 2016, 1051 HOURS.

WITH THE GROSS LACK OF JOBS AND COST OF GROCERY MASS "DISORDER" WON'T STAY AWAY MUCH LONGER.

Disorder is the main reason individual freedom on a mass scale has never existed in the history of man until the USA and its bill of rights came along. And the only way individual freedom can exist is as a byproduct of first having a genuine true free market place economy. Not the other way around.

The reason is except for harsh brutal force only a genuine true free market place economy can keep Disorder at bay. On the surface its not so obvious but the staving and purging power of a genuine true free market place economy makes it one of the most disciplining forces on earth, and it will stop "Disorder" in its tracks.

The insane arch-evil 1938 socialist minimum wage law took away that discipline power from our USA economy, which is why our judgment, morals and everything else are shallow and corrupted. Without a minimum wage law job opportunities would be unlimited even neighbors could barter or hire each other and $5.00 would buy a week's worth of grocery.

I'm about saving this country and surviving nothing more. And it may come to this extreme. I can't tell you when mass civil disorder will visit the USA to stay, but I do know we are ripe for the plucking, and it may be a lot sooner than we think.

Possibly The Greatest Weight Control Breakthrough Of The Century

Okay, having said all of that the future of the USA is obvious. Either we repeal the insane Arch-evil 1938 socialist minimum wage law to counter disorder and peacefully save our freedom, or have no choice but to resort to a physical iron fist with harsh brutal force to counter disorder.

With no jobs and sky-high grocery cost I can safely predict that an economic collapse and mass disorder will be coming to the USA soon. Now, put that in your pipe and smoke it.
SIRMANS LOG: UPDATED 08 FEBRUARY 2016, 1030 HOURS.

CHARACTER, CHARACTER, AND NOTHING BUT CHARACTER.
To all of these dense shallow minded people that dismisses proper character to gain security and prosperity, will in the end get neither. Solid character is the only thing in life that one can truly trust, especially in this day and time, nothing else, period.

This is what our insane Arch-evil 1938 socialist minimum wage law has sunk the great USA to. Sound judgment and common sense seems to have flown the coop. I swear #@%$&#@. y'all.
SIRMANS LOG: 18 FEBRUARY 2016, 1114 HOURS.

WRITER THINKS OUT LOUD:
Seems to me since the African Americans dearly love our president any perceived disrespect may trigger an overflow backlash outing at the polls. If you get my drift, need I say more...

However, the raw cold hard fact is another liberal on the high court will speed it up, but out of control liberalism is going to soon totally destroy the USA anyway. The only thing that can possibly save the USA from total doom is to repeal our insane Arch-evil 1938 socialist minimum wage law, period.

All sound judgment and common sense is already almost totally destroyed due to this 1938 law. You have the right to disagree, but very few have the almost super natural wisdom that I have. Amen. Just looking at the judgment and common sense of millions of followers today proves my point.

I sincerely hope these followers find their pot of gold at the end of the rainbow. In reality liberalism is the protector of society and a good thing. The problem is when you have out of control liberalism like we have today.

A genuine true free market place economy keeps liberalism under control and maintains a balance. Otherwise out of control extreme liberalism or conservatism will make survival impossible. Nature and life is all about balance, without balance there can be no existence.

SIRMANS LOG: UPDATED 16 FEBRUARY 2016, 0945 HOURS.

WRITER FREDDIE L SIRMANS SR'S BASIC RULE ON SUICIDE:
As a rule people with a strong survival instinct don't commit suicide. That is because one with a strong survival instinct places the survival of self, love ones, and future generations above all else, period.

Less struggle in life means less of a survival instinct, and vice-versa. Some constructive struggle must be instill at a very young age or the window may get closed forever.

Example:

Possibly The Greatest Weight Control Breakthrough Of
The Century

If a child has not learned to talk by age four the
window closes and he/she can never learn or be taught
how to talk.

Today with the young the norm seems to be a short
attention span and little staying power when faced with
a real tough challenge in my view. Myself, as long as I
can remember I hated giving up on anything. Of
course I don't mean every youngster quickly gives up.

Those with a strong survival instinct, the harder they
struggle in life the more they will be determining to
hold on to life. One has to care about more than self to
want to live when the going gets rough.
SIRMANS LOG: 14 FEBRUARY 2016, 1050 HOURS.

FROM A GUEST COMMENTER:
Maybe there is a divine reason why a neurotic
handicapped writer like Mr. Sirmans can sound a
survival stress call alarm so loud and far, only in
America. Hallelujah.
INTERRED: 10 FEBRUARY 2016, 1010 HOURS.

**ANY KIND OF TRADE WAR WILL ACT AS TRIP
WIRE TO COLLAPSE THE USA ECONOMY.**
I believe the USA economy is going to soon collapse
anyway, but any kind of trade war would instantly act
as a trip wire, and here is why? Ever since the insane
Arch-evil 1938 socialist minimum wage law the USA
economy no longer has the power or the discipline to
protect itself, the nations morals, family values, or
financial in-dependency.

The simply fact is no free nation should ever become a
permanent social and family provider if it is to survive,
period. Yet, here we are the great USA at the mercy of
an out of control obese wobbly-kneed welfare state

Possibly The Greatest Weight Control Breakthrough Of The Century

beast that is about to fall from its own weight any day now. Lord have mercy on our nation.

Government as a social and family provider on a permanent basis is like eating your seed corn or drinking your priming water. How in the hell can any free nation support a military when it supports half or more of its citizens as a first priority? #@%&$*! I love you too.

Once martial law is declared we will never see individual freedom in these United States ever again. As one with almost supernatural wisdom I figured out several years ago the only thing that can save the USA is to repeal the insane Arch-evil 1938 socialist minimum wage law, period.

As a writer my destiny is to layout the facts even if no one else believes them. I feel I have done my duty, so I am just trying to be still and remember Exodus 14:14.
SIRMANS LOG: 26 FEBRUARY 2016, 1227 HOURS.

THE LIBERAL NEWS MEDIA AND THE DEM'S ARE SECRETIVELY GLOATING
All of the predominate liberal news media and the democratic party are happy with the South Carolina republican election results, because they seem to be so sure that senator Clinton can take Trump in the general. They are secretively gloating, but no one truly knows the future, when it all boils down they may end up eating crow.
SIRMANS LOG: 20 FEBRUARY 2016, 1956 HOURS.

LAST CHANCE TO SAVE INDIVIDUAL FREEDOM IN THE USA.
One of the biggest fallacies conservatives have today is believing that cutting spending or replacing the tax

code can save the USA from total doom. It goes back to the New Deal. Once the government became a social and family provider on a permanent basis the die was cast.

Human nature means most voters are not going to bite the hand that feeds, clothes, and shelters them. When there is a gravy train more and more people are going to jump on it as time goes by. As long as government is in the role of social and family provider it doesn't matter what tax system is used government is going to take what it needs one way or another.

Repealing the 1938 minimum wage law will kick government out of the provider role and the people can take back control of their own destiny, that is the only way we can save our individual freedom, period. **SIRMANS LOG: 19 FEBRUARY 2016, 1119 HOURS.**

UP NEXT IS A CRUDE DIME STORE NOVEL I WROTE MANY YEARS AGO. IT IS NAMED " A SECOND CHANCE TO LIVE III" BY FREDDIE L SIRMANS SR.

CHAPTER   1
           Rufus Thomas was relaxed and happy on this Friday afternoon as he was taking down the   steam-table out front in the dining room, when all of a sudden he heard shots and glass breaking. Then it occurred to him like being awaken out of a dream, that someone was shooting into the restaurant. Without a second of delay, he instinctively fell to the floor.
           As he lay on the floor his mind raced back to an incident that had happened in his parking lot about a week ago. Within the last two weeks, a group of young teenagers had started using his parking lot to

make drug deals. So last week, he decided to put a stop to it.

He put his 9mm(9 millimeter semi-automatic hand gun) in his pocket and walked out to the parking lot keeping his hand in his pocket on his gun. "Hey you kids, don't y'all know this is private property?" said Rufus in a strong firm voice. One of the kids, who looked to be around 15 or 16 replied, "We have a right to be here." "Not on my property you don't. I'm telling you to get off my property right now before I call the cops."

"And if we don't?"

"That's your choice."

After swearing and grumbling, they slowly moved off down the street. After a couple of days Rufus decided to put the incident out of his mind. A voice yelling, "Mr. Thomas, Mr. Thomas are you all right?" brought him back to the present and to his feet. It was Zaporia Monique one of the two waitresses that worked for him. "Mr. Thomas, what happen? Are you all right?"

"I think so, Zaporia. Someone was shooting through the windows. I believe those kids I ran off the property about a week ago had something to do with this." Erica, the other waitress who worked at the restaurant, had come out of the kitchen to see what all of the commotion was about. "It's okay, Erica Laverne you and Zaporia go ahead and finish cleaning up, I'm going to call the police."

Bruce Allen was born in Buieville, GA. He learned early growing up in the Jimmy Carroll housing projects that you had to watch your back and fight to survive. Bruce loved his mother with all his heart but had only contempt for a father he had never met who deserted his mother before he was born.

His mother tried her best to make him go to school, but he had become more interested in making money. He had learned that money meant power, the ability to get pretty women, and the nice things in life. The youth gang in the Jimmy Carroll housing projects was called The Young Vipers. The Young Vipers' ages ranged from twelve to sixteen.

Bruce joined The Young Vipers as soon as he became eligible. By the time Bruce turned age fifteen, he was the undisputed leader of The Young Vipers. No one becomes a leader of the gang without being brutal, cunning, and savage. Some things Bruce Allen could forgive a person for, but disrespecting him was the unforgivable sin, and whoever crossed that boundary had to pay.

Growing up in the Jimmy Carroll housing projects, Bruce was no stranger to the drug business. As long as he could remember, the most successful people he knew were drug dealers. They had money, pretty women, and new cars. What else could one want? That was everything. At a very young age Bruce started in the drug business at the very bottom.

For a few dollars he would work as a lookout for the dealers and warn them if the cops were approaching. Now, he had graduated to doing a little dealing himself. Last Friday down on Mary Alice Ave., Bruce was about to close his biggest drug deal yet, when this old stooge had to come out and mess everything up. It is a perfect location for dealing drugs.

It is located off to the side where you can see who is approaching from a great distance. This is a free country, he thought. Who does that old stooge think he is going around at old disrespecting people? A few days after the incident, Bruce and a few of The Young Vipers were hanging out at Regina's Cafe. Still fuming about being disrespected, Bruce said to his second in command, "You know, Boom Boom, that parking lot down on Mary Alice Ave. is the best drug dealing location I know of.

"You're right Bruce," replied Boom Boom, "we could have that parking lot all to ourselves if nobody was in that building. I think if somebody stole a car, drove by, and shot up the place that would teach that old stooge a lesson."

"Boom Boom, I believe you're right," said Bruce.

At Buieville Police Department on Friday afternoon, Lieutenant Marvin Elder was anticipating a relaxed weekend with his family. Maybe we'll take the boat out on the lake for a few hours, he thought. Lt. Elder came from a long line of lawmen; his granddad was a deputy sheriff and two of his uncles were policemen. But his father didn't want any part of law enforcement. His father became a fire fighter.

After over eighteen years on the Buieville Police Department, Lt. Elder was nearing retirement. He started off as a foot patrolman in and around the Jimmy Carroll housing projects, which is one of the roughest neighborhoods in the city. Over the years, he served in the Traffic Division, Detective Division, Internal Affairs Division, and NARC. Division. Then about a year ago, they picked him to head up the new Youth Gang Division.

Lt. Elder was in the process of finishing up his daily reports, when his secretary Carolyn Laverne yelled, "Lt., pick up line two."

"This is Lt. Marvin Elder, may I help you?"

"Lt. Elder, this is Rufus Thomas. I operate The Harlem Garden Restaurant at 1401 S. Mary Alice Ave. We just had a drive by shooting down here."

"Was anybody hurt? "asked Lt. Elder.

"Fortunately not, I was the only one out front in the dining area; luckily my two waitresses were back in the kitchen. Also, I hit the deck after the first blast."

"Did you see the car that did the shooting?"

"Before I hit the deck I caught a glimpse of gray, but I couldn't tell what make or model it was." "

"Do you know how many shots were fired?"

Possibly The Greatest Weight Control Breakthrough Of
The Century

"I can't be for sure. Maybe three or four shots,
everything happened so fast I just can't be for sure."

"Mr. Thomas have you had any dissatisfied
customers or disputes with anyone recently."

"Yes, as a matter of fact I believe I know who is
behind this whole thing. It began about two weeks
ago when some teenagers started what looked to me
like drug dealing in my parking lot."

"Did you call the police?"

"Maybe I should have. But you know how it is,
drugs are so bad. You know they are going to do
them; you just hope they do them somewhere else.
But last Friday afternoon I got fed up and went out
there and told them to get off my property, or I would
call the cops."

"Mr. Thomas, I need to warn you. You are
definitely risking your life confronting these gangs.
They are young, but don't let that fool you; these kids
are gang members and they will not hesitate to hurt
you. Mr. Thomas, it will take me about thirty minutes
to get down there to investigate the scene and ask you
a few more questions."

"Maybe I can track down this gang who has
started using your parking lot. But Mr. Thomas, I
suggest you take precaution, because this drive by
shooting is probably the first attack in a war on you
and your property."

While pulling into the parking lot at the Harlem
Garden Restaurant, Lt. Elder's professional trained eye
alertly surveyed the parking lot and surrounding area.

He quickly saw why someone dealing drugs
would like this location. The parking lot was located
on the side of the building with just enough shrubbery
to conceal a small group of people. It was isolated
enough to allow early warning when to co someone
was approaching. The restaurant was not very large,
it probably had a seating capacity of around fifty
people. The building and landscape were clean and
well kept.

Possibly The Greatest Weight Control Breakthrough Of The Century

Pushing through the front door, he quickly noticed the liberal use of wood grain and honey colored paneling. He sensed that he would be dealing with a very conservative individual. The color scheme was pine green, navy blue, with a few spots of burgundy. The place seemed almost regal. It definitely was no cheap greasy spoon.

He noticed a man behind the serving line. "Hello sir, I'm Lt. Elder from Buleville P.D.."

"Hello, Lt. I'm Rufus Thomas the owner of this restaurant."

Lt. Elder walked to the back wall opposite the two bullet shattered front windows. Reaching into his pocket he pulled out a small leathermen's tool, then he proceeded to dig out what looked like a 9mm slug.

He next found three other bullet holes. "Mr. Thomas, your estimation of the number of shots seems to be right," said Lt. Elder. "In all I counted four bullet holes. Mr. Thomas, I would like for you to tell me everything you can think of about the kids you ran off your property last week. Did you notice anything unusual or out of the ordinary? Did you notice any scars, any limps, speech impediment, or anything that may help to identify this gang?"

There are over fifty gangs in this city, it is almost like finding a needle in a hay stack. "I'm sorry Lt., they just seem like ordinary kids," said Mr. Thomas.

"Here is my card, Mr. Thomas, please give me a call if you think of anything later that might help me find this gang. Also, give me a call if you see anything that's out of the ordinary, like the same car going past your restaurant more than normal."

"I certainly will, thank you Lt," said Mr. Thomas.

CHAPTER 2

Marion Harris, aka Loco Harris, was one of four siblings from a middle class family. One of the many baby boomers born after WWII, his father was a postal worker and his mother was a school teacher. Young Marion was an A student because that is what his parents expected of him. After high school he enrolled in a top Ivy League school. His major was ancient history. Marion was raised in a Protestant family, but in college he was exposed to people of many different religions.

Being sort of a free spirit, Marion decided to study and experiment with different religions. Shortly after getting his undergraduate degree, Marion received a draft notice. Sure, he believed that he could have enrolled in graduate school and gotten a deferent, but he decided that he would fight for his country. A year or so later Marion was a member of The Big Red 1 fighting in the jungles of Nam (Vietnam).

During his tour in Nam, Marion manage to avoid physical injury to himself, but the stress of witnessing many of his buddies being blown to bits took a mental toll on him.

Traumatic flash backs soon started invading his dreams at night. Even after getting out of the Army and returning home, the flash backs could strike without notice. No one seems to know exactly how or when Marion acquired the nick name "Loco Harris". It is said some guy on the streets started calling him that and it stuck.

Loco never married and now spends much of his time pushing a grocery store cart around town picking up aluminum cans. Loco does get a check from SSI, SSD, or somewhere.

His sister Drunell manages his money and makes sure he always has room and board. His sister Drunell won't give him much spending money because he will drink it up in beer or let the street women talk him out of it. That is why he goes around picking up aluminum cans to get beer money.

Make no mistake about it, Loco is still an intelligent man despite his mental condition. From time to time he will clean up and eat breakfast at the

Possibly The Greatest Weight Control Breakthrough Of
The Century

Harlem Garden Restaurant. If asked, Loco likes to give
lectures on world religions that he acquired great
knowledge on during his college days. Most week day
mornings Rev. Whitehurst, Deacon Bines, Deacon
Jones and a few other retirees eat breakfast and drink
coffee at the Harlem Garden Restaurant. They all are
senior citizens and retired.

They know that Loco had tried different religions
as a young man in his college days. They liked to ask
him what he was that day, a Buddhist, a Hindu, a
Moslem, or some other religion. They also knew that
would set him off on one of his lectures. They tend
not to take him seriously and will chuckle and crack a
few harmless jokes. But, never will they be mean or
cruel, because they all love Loco.

Loco has told them that he believes in a superior
being, and it doesn't matter if it is called God, Allah,
Jehovah, or whatever name. He believes there has
to be a focal point or control point somewhere or
somehow. He believes that even our sense of logic,
which we cannot escape, had to be preprogrammed
into us by some unknown organized source in some
space and time.

He stresses that modern science is discovering
by means of supercolliders that space and time is not
fixed, and that no one knows what space and time
really means. Loco believes human beings are some
type of super, super self regenerating computers that
are programmed with logic. We all experience reality
mainly through our five senses. Who really knows, we
may have many more senses that we are not aware of.

We are chemical and electrical beings.
Everything about us operates on a chemical and
electrical basis. Even our thoughts Loco believe are
made up of electrical impulses, wave lengths, and
frequencies that are far too advanced for modern
science. Out of our five senses of sight, sound, taste,
touch and smell, far more advances have been made
in the first two.

Possibly The Greatest Weight Control Breakthrough Of
The Century

Through means of modern cameras,
transmitters, and receivers man can see and hear
what is happening anywhere on earth and far into
outer space.

Electronics have come a long way since the early
days of large vacuum tubes, super heterodyne
receivers, and crude cathode ray picture tubes. There
is some progress in extending the sense of smell.
There are a few crude devices around that can imitate
the smell of a few items on a computer screen. At
some point in our near future there will probably be a
device that will imitate the smell, touch, and taste of
anything we see on a TV screen.

Janet Thomas loved her work as a nurse at Betty
Gertrude Memorial Hospital. Ever since she was a little
girl she had wanted to help and care for people. On
Fridays Janet loved to have dinner out or have some
friends over. But it's been a while since she shared a
quiet dinner at home alone with her husband Rufus.

Janet eased her brand new, willow green and
burgundy colored vinyl top Towncar into traffic. She
was accustomed to the thirty minute drive to their
ranch style home on Debra Marie Drive in Woodgate
Heights. As the town car begin to cruise, Janet
thought back to when she was twenty-years old. Then
Janet Brown, she attended Walter Bernard Community
College in San Diego. She remembered, through her
best friend Minnie Martin, she was introduced to a
young Navy Petty Officer named Rufus Thomas.

At first he seemed too serious for her taste, but
slowly she realized it was a facade to cover up his
real shyness. Underneath he had a genuine dry wit
sense of humor. As Debra Marie Drive came into view,
it brought Janet back to the present.

She checked her watch as she slowed the
Towncar and turned right onto Debra Marie Dr. The

time was five P.M. She was expecting her husband Rufus to arrive home around five thirty.

Leroy Jackson and Rufus Thomas had been friends ever since their high school days. Not a week went by that they didn't go fishing, bowling, play a game of chess, or do something together. Leroy's wife Patricia hated Rufus' political views. Leroy's political views tended to be moderate, but his wife Pat was a true bleeding heart liberal.

Pat was always telling him, "For the life of me, Leroy, I don't see why you like to hang around with that damn Rufus Thomas. I believe he is some kind of extremist rightwing nut or something. Always blaming everything on big government and the welfare state. How the hell does he think poor people and the homeless are going to survive without welfare and food stamps. I can't pay my bills as it is. I'm down to my last dollar. I sure hope they hurry up and call my number on the lottery."

Leroy enjoyed their friendship. Most of what Rufus said went in one ear and out the other. But Rufus was right about welfare and the social programs destroying the family and the extended family unit in this country.

Before pushing the key pad buttons to arm the security system and lock the front door, Rufus decided he best take Lt. Elder's advice on being cautious. He didn't always carry his handgun on him, but until this gang was caught, he planned on being prepared to defend himself at all times. He put his 9mm in his pocket and locked up.

As he merged his Silverado into traffic heading home, he thought every American should thank God they lived in a country with the freedom to bear arms, it is the rare exception, not the rule. Liberals are spouting the big lie when they say it would be safer with no guns. The real threat to our freedom and safety is not the criminal with a gun, he is only doing what he is allowed to do.

The real threat to our freedom and safety is the shallow minded liberals who allow creeping socialism to prevail. The main reason the founding fathers enacted the second amendment was not for hunting and personal protection, but as a last resort to save individual freedom from an all powerful government out of control. The fact is, there is no way we could have and continue to keep the freedoms we take for granted in this country without the freedom to possess arms. It was almost six p.m. when Rufus eased his Silverado into his carport.

After quietly letting himself in the carport door, he heard the pleasant voice of his wife saying, "Hello dear."

"Hello," said Rufus walking over to the counter near the sink where she was making a salad. Rufus gave his wife a quick kiss on the lips. "Janet," said Rufus, "a bad thing happened at the restaurant today. We had a driveby shooting."

"Oh my God! Why would anybody want to do that?", she moaned.

"I can't be a hundred percent sure, but I believe some kids I ran off the property about a week ago had something to do with it. I told Lt. Elder from the Buieville Police Dept. about the kids I ran off the property, and he seems to think they belong to one of the youth gangs operating in the city. Lt. Elder also believes the gang has declared war on me and my property."

"Rufus, you know I have asked you in the past to relocate your business out of that god forsaken area, you see how the surrounding neighborhoods have changed in the last few years."

"Gang or no gang, I am not going to let a group of kids run me off my property."

"But sweetheart, promise me you will at least consider relocating."

"Okay; I promise."

Possibly The Greatest Weight Control Breakthrough Of
The Century

"Good, said Janet. "Now you go ahead and clean up; I'm preparing us a nice candle light dinner."

As the shower water sprayed over his body, Rufus let his mind drift back to when he was a young Navy Seaman stationed at San Diego. The Navy had trained him to be a cook, but on his off-duty time he decided to take English 101 at Walter Bernard Community College.

There he got to know a young lady in his English class named Minnie Martin. At a party, Minnie introduced him to Janet Brown. At first, he thought Janet was too much of the party type for him, but he soon realized she was one of the most selfless people he had ever known.

She loved her friends, but they would never take the place of a stable home life. They got engaged, and a year later they were married. The aroma of Janet's home cooking brought him back to the present. Once they sat down to the candle light dinner and the blessing was said, Rufus thought just how much he had to be thankful for.

He had a beautiful and charming wife, a lovely daughter, Freddy Mae, who had finished college and had a career of her own as a computer programmer, and most of all he still had his life, health, and strength. Hearing Janet say, "How do you like the food Rufus?" brought him out of his deep thoughts.

"Sweetheart, it tastes great, you know how I just love your down home cooking."

After the meal they moved to the sofa in the den. They sat side-by-side on the sofa with Janet leaning gently against his chest. As they listened to their favorite oldies, Rufus gently stroked and caressed Janet's neck and shoulder area. Every now and then he would kiss her gently.

As time passed, the kisses became regular, then, more regular and passionate, still, more regular and passionate, releasing his embrace, he gently lead her to the bedroom. Later as they lay in each others arms totally spent, they told each other how much they

loved each other. Relaxing in bed after making love,
Rufus liked to express his political philosophy as long
as Janet would stay awake.

Without a reply sometimes, he would talk for
thirty minutes or more. "You know, Janet," said
Rufus, "when I see young kids committing all of these
crimes. Sure, you have to blame them primarily, but
it goes much deeper. The real blame is the welfare
state and the parents. All throughout history, the male
carried out discipline in the home until within the last
fifty years.

"Before fifty years ago this country never had a
problem with family values or ill-raised youngsters.
Then around fifty years ago, welfare and the social
programs took over the role of ed to provider and
daddy, without enforcing discipline. The first thing the
welfare and social provider did was demand that no
man could live with his family if they received
government aid.

That order drove off the one that had maintained
family values and discipline all throughout history.

"With welfare and social programs being the real
provider, the on hand female became only a stand-in
provider. Both of these new providers failed to carry
out the first duty of being a provider. That primary
duty was to maintain family discipline and values.
With raising young men, some women can be tough
and do a good job, but most can't or won't do the job.

Now, with the welfare and social program
tentacles extending all throughout this society, true
family discipline and family values in most cases are
something from the past. That is the cause of our
present state. Most of the kids in these gangs have
never had any real discipline. These kids have never
been conditioned to fear real punishment or
consequences for improper behavior.

"The only way to bring back the strong family
and extended family system is for the government to
wean itself out of the role of uncle sugar daddy. It's
only since the big government sugar daddy booted the

man, for the most part, out of the provider role that
so many of our young men are being lost to drugs and
violence.

"All that is necessary for us to solve our social
problems is for the government to get out of people's
lives as much as possible. Sure, there will be
hardship and suffering, but it has to be a natural
selection process, otherwise any do-good human
tinkering is only going to compound the problem and
make it worse.

"Another thing, is all of this hollering about jobs
going overseas. What's missing here is the jobs are
being driven overseas by big government, high health
cost, high taxes, environmental laws, and other big
government mandates.

"It's a matter of survival, no business can
compete and survive unless it makes a profit. There
must be something an ordinary citizen can do to make
a difference. Janet, you know, I think I'll try writing a
book. Janet, said Rufus a little louder. zzzzz, zzzzz,
zzzzz.

"Oh well, it was a good idea anyway," said Rufus
as he turned over on his left side, his favorite sleeping
position.

Tonight he was sure he would sleep like a baby.

Bruce Allen was age sixteen, and his mother Miss
Gracie Bell Allen thought he was in school everyday.
Sure, Bruce would leave home every school day
morning; but instead of going to school he would
spend the day playing basketball and at his girl
friend's LaTonya's house. LaTonya was on welfare, but
you wouldn't know it because she lived in a nice home
in a nice neighborhood.

LaTonya had just turned eighteen years old and
had two kids. Bruce's favorite hangout was Regina's
Cafe. Miss Felicia Regina, the lady that owns the cafe,
would sometimes get her niece LaTonya to come

down and help her out at the cafe. A little over a year
ago, Bruce started trying to talk to LaTonya, but she
wouldn't have anything to do him because she felt he
was too young for her.

A few months later, some guy started giving
LaTonya a hard time. After a while Bruce walked up
to the guy and said in a low but strong, firm tone of
voice, "Listen buddy, I'm going to ask you only one
time to leave the lady alone." The guy just stared at
Bruce for several seconds, then said, "So that's the
way it is?"

"That's the way it is," replied Bruce. The guy
said he didn't want any trouble and left.

About a week later, LaTonya invited Bruce over
to her house. Now over a year later Bruce and
LaTonya are still seeing each other. Bruce tells her he
loves her and wants to buy her a car and some of the
finer things in life. After spending most of the day
with LaTonya, Bruce, Boom Boom, and a few other
gang members were scheduled to meet that evening
at Regina's Cafe for an important meeting.

Later that evening, Bruce told the gang members
that he didn't want to kill the old stooge, he just
wanted to drive him out of business and teach him a
lesson. "Bruce, you must be getting a little soft. This
guy is armed and dangerous," said Boom Boom.

Bruce thought that it may be only a matter of
time before he would have to put Boom Boom in his
place. "Okay," said Bruce, one last time, "Everyone is
expected to have two cans of spray paint. We will
arrive at the building in groups of three and leave in
groups of three. The job shouldn't take over five
minutes. The strike time is ten o'clock. Any
questions? No questions? Then I'll see you guys
tonight."

One advantage of being a long time cop is you
have time to develop a lot of information sources.

Possibly The Greatest Weight Control Breakthrough Of
The Century

Monday morning Lt. Elder logged out to some of the
roughest neighborhoods in the city. The first stop on
his list was the Jimmy Carroll Housing Project.

Before leaving, he decided to give his secretary
Carolyn Laverne some last minute instructions.
"Carolyn, I want you to check with the record section
and see if they have any reports of gray cars being
stolen within the last week. If so, find out who found
it and any information they have on it."

"Yes sir, I will take care of that right away."

"I'll be out of the office all morning, but I should
be back around noon.

"I'll have my portable in case I have to be
reached in an emergency."

"Yes sir." It had been quite awhile since Lt. Elder
had visited the Jimmy Carroll Housing Project.

His mind raced back to about thirty years ago
when he was a young man. He remembered growing
up in the Little Miami section not very far from the
Jimmy Carroll Housing Project. Back then the projects
were a very decent and respectable place to live. As a
senior in high school, he used to play sand-lot football
and date girls in the projects.

They had a fine community center and basketball
courts. But like a lot of housing projects around the
country, it has degenerated because of crime and
drugs. To keep from completely losing it to crime and
drugs, the Buieville Police Dept. located a precinct
station there and started foot patrols.

He was brought back to the present as the five
story white brick buildings came into view.

Lt. Elder decided to park in front of the office but
not because he had any intention of going inside. He
was sure he still had a couple of long time contacts
still around. Since it was about nine a.m., there was
hardly anybody outside standing around. That suited
him fine because a lot of people were suspicious of
anyone talking to a cop for any reason.

Lt. Elder decided to try Littlejohn's apartment to
see if he was home. After reaching Littlejohn's

apartment, he pulled the screen door back and gave
three loud, quick raps on the door.

After a few seconds, he thought he heard a slight
movement inside. Then after waiting several more
seconds, he again gave three loud, quick raps. This
time he was sure he definitely heard someone
approaching the door. Then a voice barely audible
from the inside said, "Who is it?"

"Lt. Elder."

"Who?"

"Lt. Elder," he said much louder.

"Just a minute." After what seemed like a full
minute, a very small man cracked the door about six
inches. "What can I do for you Lt.?" As Lt. Elder
looked at Littlejohn he wondered what motivation, or
lack of motivation causes people to throw away their
life. Littlejohn stayed away from crack and the hard
drugs, but as Lt. Elder peered at his face and eyes he
could see that cheap wine and rot gut liquor had
certainly taken its toll.

"Littlejohn, I would like to come in and talk to
you for a couple of minutes," he said.

Littlejohn opened the door wide and stood aside.
Lt. Elder strode inside a few feet, then pivoted around
to face Littlejohn.

"Littlejohn, I want to know what the word on the
street is if any, about a driveby shooting on the
Harlem Garden Restaurant last week." lips.

"The word is, it was one of the young gangs,"
said Littlejohn.

"Do you have any names?"

"No, that's all I've heard on it."

Lt. Elder reached into his pocket and pulled out
a clip of bills and slid off a couple of twenties and told
Littlejohn, "I want names."

"Give me a couple of days," said Littlejohn.

"Here is my card; give me a call the minute you
get a name."

Leaving the Jimmy Carroll Housing Projects Lt.
Elder then made a couple more contacts. The time

was around noon so he decided to pick up some fried
rice, sweet and sour pork, a couple of egg rolls and
head on back to the office.

Rufus used to keep the Harlem Garden
Restaurant open until 9 o'clock at night during the
week and until 11 o'clock on Friday and Saturday
nights. But about a year ago, he started closing
around three thirty in the afternoon Monday through
Thursday and nine p.m. on Friday and Saturdays
because his older customers didn't like to come out at
night due to crime.

Since the driveby shooting, Rufus made sure he
was armed most of the time. He was constantly on
the alert for any sign of trouble, but so far everything
was quiet and normal around the Harlem Garden
Restaurant. Rufus wanted to finish cleaning up and
close on time this afternoon because Monday nights
was his church league's bowling night.

Five members from their church made up their
bowling team. The five members were Rufus Thomas,
Leroy Jackson,
Brenda Johnson, Danny Hebert, and Freddie Lee Jr.
Rufus would usually pick up Leroy and they would
meet the others at the bowling alley at 8 p.m. After
Rufus finished watching the six o'clock news and
Crossfire, he decided to go pick up Leroy and head to
the bowling alley.

Pulling up at Leroy's house Rufus got out and
rang the door bell. Rufus thought people who pulled
up to a person's home and sit there blowing the horn
were displaying laziness and ill manners. Why distract
or wake up the whole neighborhood?

Someone from inside the house said, "Who Is
it?"

"Rufus."

"I'm coming," said Leroy. By the time Rufus got
back in the Silverado, Leroy was coming out the front

door. "How is it going, Rufus? "said Leroy as he
climbed in the passenger side of the Silverado.

"Doing pretty good; how about you?"

"I think I'll make it." Rufus backed the Silverado
out and headed toward the bowling alley.

"Leroy," said Rufus, "do you think any one race
is more intelligent than others?"

"I never thought much about it, but I don't think
so," said Leroy.

"I don't think so either, but I do believe there
might be a cultural factor that affects motivation.

" I believe motivation affects one's intelligence
and achievement more than anything else in life, but
it is almost always ignored. In every race there will
be a smart high range and a dumb low range of
intelligence. Everyone can learn to be more
intelligent, some just have to study and work at it
harder. This is when motivation is all important.

"The big question is, why are some people highly
motivated and others not motivated at all? Some
cultures seem to highly motivate its members,
whereas other cultures don't seem to motivate its
members at all. In many cases, the more normal and
contented one is, the less motivated one is. As a rule,
those searching for love and approval are the most
motivated and highest achievers of all. In my view
the most motivated of all are insecure individuals with
a need to love or be loved."

"Rufus," said Leroy, "will you do me a favor?
Ask me if I care, it's all nonsense." Rufus didn't reply
as he turned the Silverado into the bowling alley
parking lot.

Inside the bowling alley, Rufus and Leroy
greeted the other players who were waiting on their
arrival. Their team managed to beat the Harrington
All-stars, one of the toughest teams in the league.
After saying good-by to two of the younger players,
me onl Danny Hebert and Freddie Lee Jr. Brenda
Johnson, the nurse and only female member of the
team, walked with him and Leroy back to his truck.

Possibly The Greatest Weight Control Breakthrough Of The Century

Saying good-by to Brenda, Rufus then dropped Leroy off and headed home to Janet. Once home and showered Rufus climbed into bed.

"Are you awake Janet?" said Rufus.

"Yes Rufus, I was just about to doze off, but I am fully awake now." They snuggled together in each others arms, gently kissing and anticipating, but not rushing to that distance, slowly approaching, then faster, still faster explosive ecstasy.

When Rufus arrived at the Harlem Garden Restaurant the following morning, he could hardly believe his eyes. Someone had scrawled racial graffiti all over his building. After he got inside Rufus immediately called Lt. Elder. He was told Lt. Elder didn't get in until 8 a.m., but he would get in touch as soon as he arrived.

Rufus was back in the kitchen preparing breakfast when the phone ring about eight fifteen.

"Harlem Garden Restaurant," said Rufus.

"This is Lt. Elder, may I speak to Mr. Thomas?"

"This is he."

"I got a message you wanted me to get in touch with you?"

"Yes, I wanted to report that last night somebody scrawled racial graffiti all over my building."

"Mr. Thomas, most likely it was that same gang that did the drive by shooting. Mr. Thomas give me a couple of days; I'm going to step up the effort. I promise you I'm going to find that gang and bring them to justice."

"I sure hope you find them soon," said Rufus.

"Mr. Thomas, I'll let you know the minute anything turns up." After Lt. Elder hung up, Rufus decided to call his friend Leroy Jackson.

The phone rang about three times, then a female voice said,

Possibly The Greatest Weight Control Breakthrough Of
The Century

"Hello."

"Hello Pat. This is Rufus. Is Leroy in?"

"Yes, he's out back. Hold on, I'll go get him."

After about a minute a male voice said, "Hello."

"Hello Leroy, this is Rufus, how are you today?"

"I'm doing pretty good. I was out back doing some work on my lawn mower."

"That damn gang struck again last night," said Rufus.

"What happened?"

"They spray painted and scrawled racial graffiti all over my building."

"That's terrible," said Leroy.

"I called Lt. Elder, and he promised me he was going to step up the effort and catch this gang and bring them to justice."

"I know you will be glad," said Leroy.

"You know Leroy, I've already written one letter to the editor, and I'm going to write another one today."

"Rufus, do you really think it will make any difference?"

"Leroy, I think it will.   I'm saying things that somebody needs to say about all of this big government and the welfare state."

"Ain't nothing going to change," said Leroy.

"Leroy, I believe somebody must speak out on the destruction that is being done to this country. I've decided to write a book about the dangers of the welfare state and social spending."

"Who are you going to get to publish it?" asked Leroy.

"I don't know, I may have to publish it myself. By the way Leroy, would you like to go fishing with me this Saturday evening at Grassy Pond?"

"Yes, I don't have any other plans."

"Good, I'll leave the restaurant early and let Erica and Zaporia close up. Leroy, I see some customers coming in, got to go now, I will talk to you later."

CHAPTER 3

On this Friday morning Loco Harris settled in his
chair near the Christian retirement group. Reverend
Whitehurst said,
"Loco, what religion are you today?"
Loco replied, "Guys, I first must stress that I'm
not really a religious man anymore. Everything I tell
you is strictly from a secular point of view. I must say
that I do believe in a divine power, or superior being.
You can call him God or whomever."
" How can you believe in God and not obey the
bible?" said Deacon Jones. Loco didn't answer the
question.
"You see," said Loco, "The countries of India and
China, both with populations over a billion people
contain major religions with more than one God. The
main religion in China is Buddhism, and the main
religion in India is Hinduism."
"You call them religions, as far as I'm concern
those people are all going straight to hell," said
Deacon Bines.
Loco ignored the comment and continues with
his lecture, "No matter what religion one is they all
stress avoiding thinking only of oneself. One needs to
believe in something bigger than himself. As a rule
the less selfish one is the more thankful, contented,
and happy one is.
"If one's life is unhappy and unfulfilled, the
secret is to serve God and do for others. The biggest
secret to happiness of all is to treat all people as well
as you would like to be treated, no matter how they
treat you In return. The downside to that is it is
extremely hard to treat someone well that treats you
badly, but the few that truly can, reaches a spiritual
plateau unsurpassed. The few that can truly refuse to
hate their enemies reaches a supernatural spiritual
peace that nothing can take away.

Possibly The Greatest Weight Control Breakthrough Of
The Century

"From a spiritual point of view if you speak to
someone and he won't speak back, don't feel insulted
or angry, the problem is with him, not with you. In
order to remain a good and decent person you must
try to handle every situation in a good and decent
manner. Over time one mean and unfriendly
individual can make you just like him if you play the tit
for tat game. Lastly, there is the old biblical truth that
we reap what we sow."

LaTonya couldn't wait to get home to watch her
favorite soap opera, "As The Earth Spins." She had
helped her aunt Regina at her cafe all morning. She
knew Bruce was probably playing basketball most of
the day at one of the basketball courts in the Jimmy
Carroll Housing Projects.

A dilemma was haunting her on whether to tell
Bruce that Boom Boom had made a pass at her. Boom
Boom had come on to her that morning at Regina's
Cafe. Boom Boom had told her that he didn't know
what she saw in Bruce; why didn't she give a real man
a chance. Like himself. She told Boom Boom she
wouldn't have anything to do with him if he was the
last man on earth.

She knew if she told Bruce there would be a fight
or even worse. She prided herself on being able to
handle men. She reasoned that unless Boom Boom
became too persistent or started harassing her, she
would just keep quiet on the whole matter. She had
told Bruce that she should be home by two o'clock

After playing basketball most of the day, Bruce
checked his Timex. It was two thirty; he figured
LaTonya should be home by now. He told his
teammates that would be his last game.

Bruce said farewell to the guys and left walking
to LaTonya's house. Bruce thought back to last
Monday night. He would like to scare the old stooge

that runs the Harlem Garden Restaurant off that
property, but he didn't want to kill him.

He had decided to spray paint the racial graffiti
on that building to keep up the pressure. With the
neighborhoods changing all around a lot of the older
business owners had already been scared off because
of the high crime rate. He still believed that with
enough pressure, the Harlem Garden Restaurant owner
would pull out too.

As LaTonya's house came into view, Bruce
thought LaTonya was a nice catch. Even with two kids,
she almost graduated from high school. She often
talked about getting her high school G.E.D. Bruce
was sure she was going to do it too. He had made it
to the tenth grade, but by all practical means he had
quit school.

Being only sixteen, he couldn't marry her now
even if she would agree to marry him. He had
nothing to offer her. He couldn't take care of her.
He felt fortunate because he was sure LaTonya loved
him. He felt some way, somehow he would someday
marry her. He would buy her a car, jewelry, furs and
other nice things. She was about five eight and
weighed around one hundred and forty lbs. with a
superb figure. She was very neat and clean. She
tried to hide it, but he knew secretly she was very
ambitious.

He knew she would never stay on welfare very
long. Deep down, Bruce sometimes wondered why
she put up with him.

He decided she really did love him. Bruce smiled
as he reached out to ring her door bell. He noticed
one of the curtains being pulled to one side
immediately after that, LaTonya opened the door.
"Hello, LaTonya," said Bruce.

"Hello, Bruce, are you doing all right today?"

" I'm doing pretty good." LaTonya stood to the
side as Bruce strode into the living room. He sat on
the sofa and LaTonya came over and sat beside him.

Bruce gave her a long French style kiss. "How did your day go, LaTonya."

"It went okay, how about yours?"

"I played basketball in the projects most of the day."

"Bruce, your mother thinks you are attending school. Good as you play basketball, you should go to school and play on the varsity. I'm sure you could get a scholarship to go to college."

"I don't know, LaTonya," said Bruce.

"Bruce, I've already started studying for my high school G.E.D. I hope to test before the end of the year, and if I pass I plan to enroll at Buieville Community College around the first of next year. I plan on getting my L.P.N. Degree."

Bruce leaned over and started French kissing her. Between kisses she whispered to Bruce, "My mother is keeping the kids, we have the whole afternoon to ourselves."

Friday morning Lt. Elder had planned on staying in his office and catching up on his paper work. Around eight thirty, his secretary, Carolyn Laverne, brought him a list of all the cars that had been stolen and recovered within the last two weeks.

On the list was a gray Honda Accord. He immediately picked up the phone and dialed Captain Eric Boyd, in charge of the Traffic Division.

"Hello, this is Captain Boyd Traffic Division."

"Eric, this is Marvin Elder over in the Youth Gang Division. I need some information on a gray Honda Accord that was stolen and recovered last week."

"Sure Marvin, I remember the car. We lifted several sets of fingerprints of that car. Let me transfer you to Mrs. Veronica Register, she will give you all the information we have on it."

"Hello, this is Mrs. Register, may I help you?"

"Yes, this is Lt. Elder over in Youth Gang
Division. I need some information on a gray Honda
Accord that was stolen and recovered last week."

"Just a minute, Lt., I need to bring up that file on
the computer. Okay, what do you need to know?"

"First, I would like to know where was it stolen
from."

"It was stolen from Eugene Sharpe's used car
lot."

"Where was it found."

"It was found on Sirmans' Drive near the Jimmy
Carroll Housing Projects."

"Thank you very much, Veronica, I believe that's
all I will need. Hold it," said Lt. Elder, "just one last
thing, do you know who found the car?"

"Yes, a young patrolman named Douglas
Roosevelt on the graveyard shift. That's Captain
Anthony Fuller's shift."

"I'm sure that will do it, Veronica, have a nice
weekend."

"Same to you Lt." After hanging up, Lt. Elder
thought about where the car was found. In almost all
cases wherever a stolen car is found, the culprit or
culprits live in that general area. He would ask his
information sources the names of all gangs operating
in and around the Jimmy Carroll Housing Projects. Lt.
Elder decided instead of waiting until Monday he
would go down to the Jimmy Carroll Housing Projects
and see if he could find Littlejohn.

He knew Littlejohn could give him a list of the
gangs operating in that area. He grabbed his
portable and decided to leave for the Jimmy Carroll
Housing Projects. "Carolyn;" said Lt. Elder to his
secretary, "I shouldn't be out of the office very long,
I'm going out to the Jimmy Carroll Housing Projects."

"Yes sir."

"I have my portable with me in case I have to be
located in an emergency."

"Yes sir."

Possibly The Greatest Weight Control Breakthrough Of The Century

When Lt. Elder arrived at the projects he decided to park near the office building as usual. He was hoping since it was before noon Littlejohn would still be home. He walked up to Littlejohn's front door and gave about three knocks. After a few seconds he heard movement inside.

"Who is it?" came a voice from inside.

"Lt. Elder."

"Just a minute." After what seemed like a full minute, Littlejohn opened the door.

Lt. Elder strode past him into the living room. "Littlejohn, I was hoping you would be in, I won't take but a few minutes of your time."

"Okay," said Littlejohn.

"Littlejohn, I have reason to believe the gang I am looking for is in this area." Lt. Elder got out his notepad and said,

"Littlejohn, I need the names of every gang operating in this area."

"There is a Latin gang, but I can't remember its name. There is the Young Vipers, and a little farther south is the Bonehead gang."

"How about the other gang, the Young Vipers?"

"The Young Vipers are mostly kids Lt. Some of them are as young as twelve or thirteen. The leader Bruce Allen is real mean, but seems to have some honor about himself. The real valueless one is his second in command Boom Boom. Boom Boom is the type that will take both your money and your life and feel no remorse."

Lt. Elder reached into his left pocket and pulled out a clip of bills, slid off five twenties and thanked Littlejohn.

"One other thing Littlejohn, where can I find Bruce Allen and the other leaders. Where do they hang out?"

Littlejohn thought for a minute. "Lt. there are two places Bruce Allen likes to hang out. Almost everyday, sometimes during the day, you will find him playing basketball on one of the courts here in the projects. The other place he like to hang out at is, Regina's Cafe down on S. Mary Alice Ave."

On his way back to his office Lt. Elder decided he would wait until Monday to follow up on those names. He believed one of those gangs was the one he was looking for.

Saturday, Rufus told Erica to close up the restaurant. He was taking off early to go fishing. At home, Rufus was deciding on what gear and fishing equipment to use. He decided to take along his spinning reel just in case the biting was slow. Then he might decide to do a little casting for bass using plastic worms. But today, he planned on fishing for bream or blue gill, a very good pan fish.

Rufus decided to use a light limber eight-foot long bamboo cane pole. That would allow him very good wrist action to pitch his bait from spot to spot while the boat slowly trolled the lake. The minute he got a bite, he would quietly anchor down.

If he didn't continue getting bites, he would start back trolling.

He decided on a number five blue steel hook that would bend without breaking.

He also decided to use a fifteen pound test line with a B.B. shot lead weight, about six inches from the hook and use a small slim line cork so there would be very little resistance when the fish bit and pulled on the hook. He also decided he would take along both crickets and red wigglers for bait. Finally, making sure there were at least two safety vests on board, he decided to give the fifteen foot bass master one last going over. Then he hooked her up to the Silverado.

Before leaving his house, he called Leroy to let him know that he was on his way. After leaving Leroy's house, they pulled into Alfred Myers Bait and Tackle Shop. They each purchased about fifty crickets and a small container of red wigglers. Now, finally,

they were on their way. As he turned into the Old
Stockton Road leading out of the city, Rufus smiled to
himself and wondered if Sarah Whitlock still lived on
this road.

He remembered years ago she was his first
employee at the Harlem Garden Restaurant. She fell
in love and married a rich undertaker, then he made
her quit to take care of their eventually ten kids.
They used to live in a nice colonial style home with
bay windows on this road. He watched Leroy light up
and take a long drag on his cigarette.

He often thanked God he found the strength
several years ago to quit that costly stupid health
snatching habit. But he guessed we all have a
weakness for something.

"Leroy," said Rufus, "what do you think about
people always complaining that they can't find any
jobs?

"I don't think there are very many good jobs
left," said Leroy, "all we got is jobs flipping
hamburgers or some other minimum wage job.

"What I really think," said Rufus," is all of this
crying about no jobs is a red herring or some other
phony excuse. Just think about it, we have millions of
illegal aliens in this country easily finding work. But
somehow, poor Americans can't find work.

The availability of hard, tough work is the bait
that is drawing the illegals to this country. If it was
not for our welfare state, those now on welfare would
have to do hard tough work, and there would be no
jobs left to draw millions of illegals to this country. As
for those minimum wage jobs, I have worked them
and feel that anyone that has to work will take any job
he can get until he can do better.

"One other thing is, this complaining about rich
people making money. Attacking the rich is the first
thing a dictator or socialist does. They try to falsely
blame the rich for all shortcomings. That way they
can distract and mislead the uninformed, while they
promote their own power grabbing agenda. Balance is

the key. We need a strong middle class. Nobody poor is going to give anybody a job, so it stands to reason the more rich people we have and produce the more jobs we all will have. You can't get blood out of a turnip. Somebody has to have money to pay those that don't have any, otherwise nobody will have money to pay those that don't have any, like in a socialist system."

"Rufus," said Leroy, "don't miss your turn, next right."

"Okay, I won't. Let me say this last thing and I'll get off this subject. There is no shame in doing hard, tough work as long as one has the freedom and opportunity to better himself. But we will never get Americans to do hard, tough work as long as we have a welfare state like ours. There will always be some excuse not to work."

As they were pulling up to Grassy Pond, Leroy said, "I sure hope we catch a big mess of fish. There is nothing better on a Saturday night than a big bowl of cheese grits, coleslaw, sliced onions, deep fried fish, and hush puppies."

Once they got the fourteen foot bass master unloaded, they decided to slowly troll around the east side of the lake first.

They decided to start off using cricket first. Rufus took the front seat. He positioned the foot pedal for comfort to best guide and direct the boat. As the bass master named Yvette slowly eased through the water, Rufus used a slight wrist action with his light eight foot pole to pitch his cricket from one spot to the next.

They were about a hundred yards out in the lake when all of a sudden a blue gill hit his bait so hard his bamboo cane pole bent almost to the breaking point. As Rufus finally snatched the blue gill out of the water and let the fish slowly swing back to his open left palm, he then eased it into the live-well.

Possibly The Greatest Weight Control Breakthrough Of
The Century

One of the challenges of bringing in a big blue
gill is they will turn sideways on you, then a pound
and a half fish will pull like an five pound bass.

"Leroy," said Rufus softly, "ease out the anchor."
When Rufus snatched the blue gill out of the water, he
saw a clear, watery liquid streaming from the fish. He
knew instantly this was their lucky day.

He realized it must be a full moon and the fish
were on bed, meaning the fish would be in large
groups and the males would be fertilizing the female
eggs. He knew if it was a big bed they could catch
their allotted amount in short order, because on a
bed, you can catch them as fast as you can bait up.
Unfortunately, it was a small bed.

They caught about ten blue gills as fast as they
could throw out. Then nothing for the next fifteen
minutes. It was not long before they found another
bed. After being on the pond for a little over two
hours, they had their allotted catch, then they headed
for home. Once Rufus had dropped Leroy and his
share of the fish off, he eased the Silverado back into
traffic for the twenty minute drive to his home.

As the Silverado droned on, Rufus thought back
to when he was a young petty officer in the U.S. Navy
stationed in San Diego. Their daughter Freddy Mae
was born after he and Janet had been married a little
over a year. Both parents doted on their only
daughter. She was taught to be responsible for her
actions. She was taught to treat all people well and
decently as she would like to be treated no matter
how she was treated in return, but always defend
herself and not take any abuse. She was taught to
always look for a reason to succeed instead of
accepting any excuse for failure.

His mind came back to the present as Debra
Marie Drive loomed into view. As he turned onto
Debra Marie Drive, Rufus smiled to himself and
decided he would call his daughter when he got home.
Rufus put away his boat and secured everything.

Possibly The Greatest Weight Control Breakthrough Of
The Century

He decided to clean just enough fish for a good meal. The rest make y of the fish he placed in two one gallon plastic milk containers with the top cut off them. He then filled them with water, and placed them in the freezer. He would clean the rest later as needed.

That night, he and Janet enjoyed a supper of cheese grits, coleslaw, sliced raw onions, dill pickle, deep fried fish, and hush puppies. Afterwards, they cuddled together on the sofa in the den, and viewed one of the latest video movies.

"By the way, Janet," said Rufus, "I have managed to finish writing two chapters in my book. I have also decided on a name for it. The name will be "Why We Must Dismantle The Welfare State," by Rufus Thomas.

CHAPTER 4

It had been quite awhile since Loco had eaten breakfast at the Harlem Garden Restaurant. After Loco had settled comfortably at his usual table, one of the Christian retirement group members said, "Hey Loco, are you a Hindi today?" They knew that would launch Loco on one of his lectures. After several seconds Loco replied, "You know, way back around 1500 BC the Hindu religion was born in India.

"Hinduism is a very old religion and it has had a big influence on many other religions over the years. Hinduism is a major world religion, and it is estimated to have more than 700 millions followers, mostly in India. Like most eastern religions, Hinduism regards more of what people do rather than what they think.

"It focuses mainly on rules for behavior and conduct. They acknowledge the existence of many gods, but most individuals are primarily devoted to a single God or Goddess. Most westerners know that they have a reverence for Brahmans and cows that

prohibits them from eating beef. Their main text or
authority is the Vedas.

"I still say that is a lot of soul being lost," said
Reverend Whitehurst. cause

"Amen," said Deacon Jones.

LaTonya yelled at her two-year-old son because
he was making too much noise banging a toy upside
the wall. For Christ's sake, she couldn't hear what
Karen Parker was saying on her favorite soap opera,
"As The Earth Spins." She checked the time; it was
almost noon. She decided to boil some wieners. Her
boyfriend Bruce should be over soon and he might be
hungry.

That reminded her to check her food stamps; the
baby was almost out of milk. She would get Bruce to
run to the store and get some milk and Fruit Loops.
She put the wieners on slow cooking and returned to
the sofa to watch her soap. As she watched the
beautiful Asia Greene seduce her leading man on the,
"Youth And The Reckless," she thought back to a
couple of years ago when her stepfather had tried to
rape her.

She had to go live in Miss Louise Gardner's
Orphanage for young girls. Miss Gardner was very
strict, but she was fair.

She taught her girls to believe in themselves,
that they could be whatever they wanted to be.
Someone knocking on her front door brought her back
to the present. LaTonya walked over to the window
and slightly parted the curtains to see who it was.

It was Bruce, and she immediately opened the
door.

"Hello, LaTonya," said Bruce.

"Hello Bruce, how are you today?"

"Pretty good," said Bruce as he strode past her
and sat on the living room sofa.

Possibly The Greatest Weight Control Breakthrough Of
The Century

Bruce sat beside her on the sofa. He still found
it hard to believe that he could hold on to a charming
girl like LaTonya.

"Bruce," said LaTonya, "would you like for me to
fix you a couple of hot dogs?"

"Yes, I would like a couple of hot dogs."
LaTonya got up walked over to the refrigerator and
took out about three hot dog buns.

"Bruce, what would you like on your hot dogs?"

"Just ketchup and mustard will be fine."
LaTonya finished Id go fixing the hot dogs and
brought them and a soda to Bruce on the sofa.

"Bruce, when you finish eating I would like for you to
go to the store and get me some milk, and Fruit Loops
for the kids."

"Okay, LaTonya, I'm going to leave early today.
My mom told me to be home when she got off from
work. She wants to have a very important talk with
me." After eating his hot dogs, Bruce left for the
nearest Flash Food Minute Market about a block away.

It took him about thirty minutes to return from
the Minute Market. LaTonya made her two kids take
their daily nap, then she took Bruce's hand and gently
led him to her bedroom.

Later, as they lay talking she asked Bruce to
please get out of the gang and go back to school.
Bruce said he would think about it. Bruce checked his
Timex. "LaTonya," said Bruce, "it is almost five
o'clock I really must go. I will try to come over later
tonight."

"Okay, I will get up and walk you to the door."

When Bruce got home, his two sisters, Tasha age
fifteen and Tameka age fourteen were doing their
homework. His mom was in the bathroom. Bruce sat
on the living room sofa and started watching TV.
After about fifteen minutes, Bruce's mother Miss
Gracie Bell Allen came out of the bathroom.

"Tasha," yelled Ms. Gracie Bell, "is Bruce home
yet?"

"Yes maam, he's watching TV in the living room."

Possibly The Greatest Weight Control Breakthrough Of
The Century

"Bruce," yelled Miss Gracie Bell, "I want to talk
to you in your room."

"Yes maam." As Bruce ascended the stairs to his
room, he wonders what it was that his mother wanted
to talk to him about that seemed so important.

He decided to himself that the jig was up; he
was busted.

He knew it had to be about him playing hooky
from school. As his mother stood by his room door,
he strode past her into his room and sat on the side of
his bed. His mother followed him into the room and
closed the door. "Bruce," said Miss Gracie Bell, "I
want the truth. I don't want to hear any lies. I want to
know have you been going to school every morning
when you leave here?"

Bruce thought about lying but sensed that his
mother already knew the truth. After taking longer
than necessary to answer, Bruce finally said, "No
maam."

"Where have you been going every school day?"

"I've been playing basketball here in the projects
and going to a friend's house."

"Who is this friend that you have been going to
his house instead of going to school?"

"It is a she."

"I see," said his mom. "What is her name?"

"LaTonya Smith."

"How old is she?"

"She just turned eighteen."

"I want to find out more about this LaTonya
woman, but that can wait. It was late when you got
home last night, and I decided to wait until I got off
work today to talk to you. The high school principal's
office called me yesterday afternoon, and we had a
long talk concerning you. They think you are headed
for serious trouble. They think you not only skip
school, but you are also involved in gang activity.
They feel it is only a matter of time before you will be
dealing hard drugs. Bruce, I brought you into this
world, and damn it, I will take you out of it.

Possibly The Greatest Weight Control Breakthrough Of
The Century

"Bruce, I have made my share of mistakes, but I
will not stand for this. I promise you if you stay in
this house, you are going to school. Tomorrow, I'm
going out to the school and talk to the principal. I'm
going to tell her the first day of school you miss I
want to know about it. I may have to send you to live
in the country on your Uncle Hoover Charles' farm, but
you can rest assured that if you skip school again there
will be severe consequences. Do you understand me,
young man?"

"Yes maam."

Monday morning Lt. Elder had already decided to
bring in the leaders of two gangs. He decided to go
after the Young Vipers first. The leaders of the Young
Vipers were a sixteen- year-old name Bruce Allen, and
another sixteen-year-old that went by the name Boom
Boom. Lt. Elder knew he may need extra help in
making this bust just in case things turned sour. Lt.
Elder decided two other sergeants in the youth gang
division may not be enough manpower.

He decided to bring in four additional uniformed
officers for back up. One of the uniformed officers
was a tough battle scarred chap named Lt. Joe Walsh.
The other uniformed officers were Staff Sergeant
Roger Miller, Corporal Dana Mitchell, and Corporal
Charlie Johnson. Lt. Elder had the names of the gang
leaders, but he didn't have the slightest idea how
these kids looked.

He already had his task force organized and
ready to move, but since he didn't know how these
kids looked he needed to do a little leg work first. He
had already gotten permission from Police Chief
Jimmy Sampson to exempt members of his task force
from other duties. The Young Vipers were reported to
hang out at Regina's Cafe.

Lt. Elder told his secretary to log him out to
Regina's Cafe and from there to the Jimmy Carroll

Housing Projects. He should be back in a couple of hours. It was around nine thirty when Lt. Elder entered Regina's Cafe. There were no customers around at the time. The cooking area was behind the counter and about midway behind the counter, was a big, black eight burner gas stove with a large, smooth iron grill on the left and a large baking oven on the right.

At the far end of the counter toward the back of the diner, was what looked to be a storage room and office. Two women, who looked to be in their early thirties, seemed to ignore him and continued with their chores. Clearing his throat, Lt. Elder said, "I would like to speak to the owner."

"I am," said the lady nearest to him with a pleasant voice and ready smile as she turned around to face him. "I'm Miss Felicia Regina, owner of this establishment."

"I'm Lt. Elder from Buieville P.D." as he flashed his badge.

"Miss Regina do you know a sixteen-year-old by the name of Bruce Allen?" I have information that he and his friends come in here often.

Miss Regina looked in the direction of her employee, Miss Anna Ruth Leonard. "Anna Ruth, ain't that the name of the young man that be talking to my niece?"

"I do believe it is, Miss Regina."

"Lt. I do believe I know the young man, what he done?"

"We just need to ask him some questions," said Lt. Elder.

"How about the name Boom Boom; do you know him?"

"I don't think so." "

"Well, he's Bruce Allen's right hand man and is with him most of the time."

"You're right Lt.; the same one or two friends are with him almost all the time."

"Miss Regina, do you have a phone in the back
where there is privacy?"

"Yes, I have one back in my office."

"Miss Regina, I would like to ask a favor of you.
You don't have to do it if you don't want to."

Lt. Elder reached in his shirt pocket and pulled
out a card.

"This is the number you can reach me," he said
as he handed Miss Regina his card. "1 would like for
you to give me a call if Bruce Allen or any of his friends
come in here today. Remember you don't have to do
this if you don't want to."

"I'll give you a call Lt."

"Make sure you use the phone in back because
the call must be in complete privacy. Also, make sure
you describe the color and type of clothes they are
wearing. Before I go, may I use your phone?"

"Sure Lt., come on around behind the counter,"
as she led him back to her office. Lt. Elder called his
secretary and told her to contact him immediately on
his portable if he got a call from Regina's Cafe. It was
almost ten thirty when Lt. Elder arrived at the Jimmy
Carroll Housing Projects.

He parked in the office parking lot as usual and
made his way to Littlejohn's apartment. Once inside
Littlejohn's apartment, Lt. Elder asked him if he could
identify Bruce Allen and Boom Boom.

"Sure, I can identify both of them," said
Littlejohn. "I see Bruce Allen playing basketball here
in the projects almost every day. Boom Boom don't
care as much for basketball, but he do be on the side
line watching most of the time."

"What I would like for you to do, Littlejohn, is
monitor all of the basketball courts here in the
projects and the minute Bruce Allen or Boom Boom
shows up give me a call. Since I don't know how he
looks, make sure you give a good description of the
color and type of clothes they will be wearing." Lt.
Elder reached in his shirt pocket and pulled out one of
his cards, then reached in his left trouser pocket and

pulled out a money clip, slid off a couple of twenties
and thanked Littlejohn. Lt. Elder returned to his office
and decided to catch up on his paper work while he
wait on the expected calls.

It was almost one o'clock when Lt. Elder received
the call from Regina's Cafe. Miss Regina told Lt. Elder
that two of Bruce Allen's friends were in her place of
business. They both looked to be around age sixteen
and had on long shirts about three sizes too large.
One of the shirts was gray with sea shell like designs,
the other shirt was green with flowery designs.

"Okay guys," said Lt. Elder. "Let's go make this
bust."

Lt. Elder and the other two plain cloths
detectives from the Youth Gang Division rode in his
unmarked sedan. Lt. Joe Walsh and the other three
uniformed officers rode in two black and whites. Their
instructions upon arrival was for the detectives to go
in first and the uniformed officers to lag behind a
little. When Lt. Elder pushed open the front door, he
immediately spotted the two gang members. He
cautiously approached their table and came to a stop
directly in front of them. "Buieville P.D.," said Lt.
Elder as he flashed his badge.

"Which one of you goes by the name of Boom
Boom?"

"I do," said the youth in the gray shirt.

"I'm placing both of you under arrest for
suspicion in a driveby shooting. You have the right to
remain silent. Anything you say can and will be used
against you in a court of law. You have the right to
talk to a lawyer and have him present with you while
you are being questioned. If you cannot afford to
hire a lawyer one will be appointed to represent you
before any questioning, if you wish one. Stand up,
turn around, and place your hands behind your back."
The two youths did as they was told and showed no
resistance.

Both suspects were led outside and placed in one
of the black and whites. Lt. Elder dismissed the other

two sergeants from the Youth Gang Division plus one black and white and two corporals. He instructed Lt. Joe Walsh and the other uniformed officer in the black and white with the suspects to follow him. He wanted to stop by the Harlem Garden Restaurant on S. Mary Alice Ave.

About ten minutes after leaving Regina's Cafe, they arrived at the Harlem Garden Restaurant. After entering the restaurant, Lt. Elder asked the waitress out front to speak to Mr. Thomas.

The waitress went to the kitchen, and Mr. Thomas immediately came out front. "Hello, Lt.," said Mr. Thomas, "what can I do for you?"

"I have a couple of suspects of that driveby shooting outside.

I would like for you to come outside and see if they were the youths you ran off your parking lot."

"I would be glad to take a look." Lt. Elder led Mr. Thomas out to the black and white. Mr. Thomas leaned over to get a better view of the youths inside.

Then he walked a few feet away with Lt. Elder at his side. "The one in the gray shirt was definitely one of the kids I ran off my parking lot."

"Thank you, Mr. Thomas, we will take it from here." Lt. Elder took both youths back to the station for questioning. Boom Boom was told his fingerprints were found on the stolen car, but he denied any involvement in any driveby shooting.

He was sent to the district youth correction center in Belview, then two weeks later, he was sentenced to 4 months of boot camp. The other youth broke down during questioning and told everything and was released into the custody of his parents.

CHAPTER 5

After saying good morning on this Good Friday morning, Loco settled in his seat at his favorite table at

the Harlem Garden Restaurant. Sometimes the
Christian retirement group would engage Loco in just
pleasant small talk and let it go at that. For a while it
seemed like that was the way the   morning would go,
but then one of the group members just couldn't
resist saying, " Loco, you must be a Buddhist today I
suppose?"

"No, I am not," said Loco. " However, I must tell
you that Buddhism also is a major world religion.

"There is estimated to be over 400 millions
Buddhist followers world wide. Back in the 6th
century BC in India they believed that over long cycles
of time wisdom returned to earth and was given to a
chosen individual, that person would be known as the
Budda. In the 6th century BC in India, Siddhattha
Gautama lived a life of leisure and pleasure because
he was a member of a privileged and influential family.

"Just like today when there is very little
challenge or struggle in one's life, it leaves a void.
Gautama's life was unfulfilled, and he went in search
to try to find meaning and purpose to his life. At that
time in India the ascetic life was a long practice for
those seeking a deeper meaning to life. Guatama had
acquired five companions and followers in leading his
ascetic life, but they deserted him when he decided to
eat regularly.

"Gautama then spent a long time wandering
alone. Then one day he seated himself under a large
Bo tree by the side of the river. There he said a clear
vision came to him. There he said the keys to life
came to him. Then he arose to go teach his vision.
He found his five former followers, and after five days
he finally convinced them that he was now truly
enlightened. They then shouted and proclaimed him
as the Budda.

"The main points of Gautama's vision was that all
miseries in life is because of selfishness, and greedy
desires. Nirvana is the highest goal of the Buddhist
path, an enlightened state when the desires of greed,
hatred, and ignorance have been overcome. Buddhist

are found mostly in Asia, but almost none in India
where it was started.
    "Buddhism has greatly evolved over the
centuries. Several new sects developed in China. One
of the sects most well known is Zen. Zen is the most
popular sect found in the US."

    Rufus decided he was not going to write a large
book and that he would keep it down to around a
hundred pages. He estimated he would be finished
with his first draft in about another week. Since he
identified one of the gang members for Lt. Elder, he
felt finally this gang threat would soon be over.
    He was in a good mood so he decided to do
some writing on his manuscript.
    He decided to write about one subject that he
was truly sick and tired of. He was sick and tired of
all this damn blaming everything and everybody but
one's self in today's society.
    You can talk to anyone successful, and he will tell
you the key to success is to try and keep trying no
matter the circumstances.
    People that are always looking for something or
somebody to blame are in his view irresponsible and
dangerous. Just think about it, he thought, if one is
independent and responsible he is not going to waste
time blaming and depending on others. The surest
proof of one's dependency and irresponsibility is
wasting time and exercising in futility because
someone doesn't like or accept him. It is
irresponsible to waste time blaming others because
they don't like you.
    The fact is, if you are a good and decent person,
good and decent people are going to accept you,
otherwise they don't matter. Who cares so long as
they can't hurt you. You can't make people like you if
they don't want to, and it's dumb and shallow to
think otherwise. The same people that are always

blaming others are not doing a damn thing of substance for themselves or their fellow man.

All these years of welfare and social spending have conditioned far too many people to expect the government and others to do for them while they sit back and blame and complain. It has given far too many people a dependent mentality. They feel they are entitled to everything anybody else has without having to earn it. They try to blame and lay a guilt trip on others that prosper and earn their way instead of making their own actions produce worthy results.

It's a matter of focus. When a good ball team gets a bad call, it doesn't start focusing on the officiating but instead keeps its focus on its winning game plan. That is the same way it should be when dealing with racism. One should keep his focus on his goal and not lose focus on racism or anything negative.

It's impossible for racists or haters to destroy your mind unless you hate them back, then your own hate may end up consuming your mind and soul. If you get down into the gutter to settle a dispute with someone, there is no way to come out looking sparkling clean.

Sure, there is racism in this country, and I've faced it first hand, but my focus is on becoming as physically independent and self sufficient as possible. I for one don't fear racism because this country still offers me many options to become as good or successful as anyone. I'm not soft on racism.

I am completely against racism and bigotry in any form. It's just that we live in a real world and it is not wise to completely ignore human nature. The fact is, as long as different races are living among one another there is going to be some racism whether people admit it or not. Many of those complaining the loudest about racism are the biggest racists of them all.

It is short sighted for a minority race to be perceived or treated special in anyway, because it divides and turns other races against them. Things like affirmative action and hate crimes on the surface may seem helpful, but in the long run they divide and cause resentment among the races.

Sure, big government can protect us now, but nothing remains the same, and sooner or later the majority race is going to get its redress.

Racism will never keep a do-for-yourself person down when he has the freedom and opportunity like in this country.

All it is is another obstacle to overcome and overcoming obstacles is what makes successful people successful. The sensible thing is to concede racism, because as long as there are different races one will have to deal with it sooner or later.

Whether it is admitted or not, every race has its share of racists.

The solution is instead of all this blaming, we need more do- for-yourself Americans like in the days before the welfare state began. A do-for-yourself person is going to be more concerned about what he is going to do for himself than what somebody else may or may not do.

One other thing, when the liberals keep chanting let's put children first, let's put children first, let's put children first, they forget about the unborn aborted children. They were our future children too. To claim the government is responsible for our children is the main reason why our society is in a complete decline. Every individual parent is solely responsible for his or her own children, not the government , nor anyone else, unless the children are legally taken from the parent.

This whole government and society is on the brink of going bankrupt and breaking up like the former Soviet Union unless something is done to save our currency from becoming worthless from out of control spending. Still, you have shallow minded liberals demagoging the issue by hiding behind children. The sad fact is, if we don't start cutting

spending and save this great nation nobody is going
to be able to help the children or anybody. Sure,
liberals care greatly about this nation and the things
they advocate, but in most cases, their care is shallow
and superficial.

Sixty years ago almost everyone was
conservative because of the hardships and struggles
to survive. Now, far too many people have become
shallow with weak survival instincts, due to big
government and social spending. It's a perception
problem. You can't get most people to see the value
of self sufficiency and tough love in today's society.
But, the facts are self sufficiency and tough love are
survival tools that could save millions of lives if a
severe calamity hit, and believe me, with the decline
of our family and moral values this nation is becoming
more and more vulnerable.

The best thing for a liberal is a little hardship and
struggle that will wake him up and open his eyes. A
little hardship and struggle will give a liberal some
depth by sharpening his survival instinct. A weak
survival instinct is why any society that has it too
easy, will eventually destroy itself. There has to be
some real, or imposed hardship and struggle in one's
life in order to build good judgment and character.

Rufus checked his watch; it was well after five,
so he decided he had better quit writing for now. He
closed up the restaurant and went on home. On
Friday nights, Rufus and Janet liked to attend all of
their local high school home football games. Tonight,
the Buieville Tigers were playing cross town rival,
Hutto High Trojans at home.

It was around seven thirty on this clear fall night
when Rufus and Janet left for the game. The sleek,
new Towncar cruised through the silent, crisp cool
South Georgia night air with the smooth grace of a
champion race horse. They arrived at Lomax Field

about ten to eight. That would give them ten minutes
to settle in their seats before game time.

Tonight, the Buieville Tigers were facing
undefeated cross town arch rival Hutto High Trojans.
At half-time, the Tigers were up fourteen to seven.
Late in the fourth quarter, the Tigers were down
twenty to twenty-one with only fifteen seconds left in
the game. On second and goal, the Tigers had just
taken their last time out with the ball on the Hutto
High Trojans' two yard line. Instead of kicking a field
goal it appears the Tigers are going to run another
play.

The referee windmills his hand to signal that time
has started. The Tigers all state quarterback Hoover
Sirmans II is under center. He drops straight back
about five yards, he looks, he looks, he looks, ten,
nine, eight, seven, six, all receivers covered, Sirmans
zooms the ball over everyone's head out the back of
the end zone. Three seconds left on the clock, the
kicking team automatically runs onto the field. Both
teams are set. The kick holder gives the signal. The
hike is good. The kick holder places the ball. The
soccer style kicker follows through and keeps his head
down, never looking up until he hears the roar of the
crowd, then he is literally mobbed. There is sheer
pandemonium as the home crowd goes wild.

Rufus still felt elated as he and Janet left the
stadium and headed for home. "Janet," said Rufus, "I
feel like celebrating a little, how about us stopping by
the Dairy Queen for some ice cream?" "That would be
nice, Rufus, I believe I will have a banana split."
There was no line so Rufus was able to drive straight
up to the drive-in station.

"May I help you?" said the speaker at the drive-
in station.

"Give me a large cup of ice cream with nuts on
top and a banana split," said Rufus.

"Will that be all sir?"

"Yes."

Possibly The Greatest Weight Control Breakthrough Of
The Century

"That will be three seventy five, drive around
please."

Rufus received his order, paid his bill, and
headed for home.

After arriving home, Rufus and Janet sat on the
sofa in the den.

Rufus put on some soft oldies music and they
enjoyed their ice cream. Later they fell asleep in each
other's arms after n some consummating the night in
perfect bliss and ecstasy.

Around three thirty, Lt. Elder and the other
officers were still on alert static. "Lt. Elder, Littlejohn
on line two," said his secretary Carolyn Laverne.

"Lt. Elder speaking."

"Lt. I have bad news, I can't figure it out, Bruce
Allen is always playing basketball everyday here in
the projects. I don't know what happened, but I
haven't seen him all day."

"Littlejohn," said Lt. Elder, "you can call it a day.
I appreciate the effort you gave it."

After hanging up from talking to Littlejohn, Lt.
Elder decided he was going to release most of the
task force. He decided to hold over two of the
uniformed officers, Lt. Joe
Walsh and Corporal Dana Mitchell. Everyone else was
dismissed. During questioning, they managed to get
some crucial information out of the youth with Boom
Boom.

They know where Bruce Allen lives, where he
supposedly went to school, where his girl friend lives,
etc. After releasing the other members of the task
force, Lt. Elder in his sedan and the two uniformed
officers in their black and white, headed for Bruce
Allen's home in the Jimmy Carroll Housing Projects. It
was after four o'clock when they arrived at Bruce
Allen's address.

Possibly The Greatest Weight Control Breakthrough Of The Century

Lt. Elder and the other two uniform officers walked up to Bruce Allen's apartment. Lt. Elder pulled the screen door back and gave three loud raps.

"Who is it?" said someone from the inside.

"The police."

A wide eyed girl opened the door immediately.

" Does Bruce Allen live here?" said Lt. Elder.

"Yes sir."

"We would like to talk to him."

"He ain't home."

"Do you know where we can find him?"

"No sir." long

As Lt. Elder and the officers walked back to their cars, "Joe," said Lt. Elder, "school has already turned out for the day. The most likely place he will be is at his girl friend's house."

Shortly thereafter they arrived at LaTonya's home on Cummings Street. As the officer's approached LaTonya's front door, Lt. Elder instructed Corporal Mitchell to go around to the back door just in case Bruce tried to skip out. When Lt. Elder knocked on the front door, they noticed a curtain near the door part slightly. Within a few seconds, a young lady opened the door about eight inches.

Past her, Lt. Elder could see a young man sitting on the sofa.

"Is Bruce Allen here," said Lt. Elder?

The young lady just stared at him for several seconds.

Finally, she said, "Yes, he is here."

"We would like to talk to him."

LaTonya opened the door wide and stood aside. Lt. Elder and Lt. Joe Walsh entered the living room.

"Are you Bruce Allen?" said Lt. Elder to the young man sitting on the sofa.

"Yes sir, I am," said Bruce Allen.

"I am placing you under arrest as a suspect in a driveby shooting. You have the right to remain silent. Anything you say can and will be used against you in a court of law. You have the right to talk to a lawyer

111

and have him present with you while you are being
questioned. If you cannot afford to hire a lawyer one
will be appointed to represent you before any
questioning, if you wish one. Stand up, turn around,
and place your hands behind your back." Bruce Allen
did as he was told and offered no resistance.

Lt. Elder used his car phone to call Rufus Thomas
at the Harlem Garden Restaurant, but he didn't get an
answer. He then called Mr. Thomas' home and his
wife said he hadn't arrived from the restaurant yet. Lt.
Elder left word for Mr. Thomas to call him at his office
as soon as he got home. Back at the station, Lt. Elder
questioned Bruce Allen about his involvement in the
driveby shooting on the Harlem Garden Restaurant.

Bruce Allen denied any involvement in the
driveby shooting or the spraying of graffiti. Around
five thirty, Rufus Thomas called. Lt. Elder asked him
if he would come down and identify another youth
that he believed was involved in the driveby shooting.
Mr. Thomas said he would be there in about thirty
minutes. Lt. Elder also called Bruce Allen's mother and
informed her of the trouble Bruce was in. She said she
would be down right away.

Upon arrival at the station, Rufus Thomas told
the desk sergeant why he was there. The desk
sergeant paged Lt. Elder to the front desk. "I'm glad
you could come down, Mr. Thomas," said Lt. Elder as
he approached the front desk.

"I'm more than glad to do whatever I can to help
bring these criminals to justice."

"Come with me, Mr. Thomas," said Lt. Elder as
he led him to a viewing room that was behind a two
way mirror.

Once inside the viewing room, Lt. Elder told Mr.
Thomas to see if the youth in the other room was one
of the youths he ran off his property.

"That's him," said Mr. Thomas, "that's the one
that did the talking."

"Are you absolutely sure," said Lt. Elder.

"Without a doubt in my mind."

Possibly The Greatest Weight Control Breakthrough Of
The Century

"Thank you very much, Mr. Thomas, you can go
now."

Lt. Elder led him back to the front desk. "Thanks
again, Mr. Thomas, for coming."

"You're welcome."

After Mr. Thomas' departure, Lt. Elder begin
making arrangements to have Bruce Allen
transported to the district youth correction center at
Belview. Lt. Elder was paged to the front desk. He
was sure it must be Miss Gracie Bell Allen, Bruce
Allen's mother. "Hello, I'm Lt. Elder. Are you, Bruce
Allen's mother?" asked Lt. Elder as he approached the
front desk.

"Yes, I'm his mother." and I

"Miss Allen, we are sure your son is guilty. We
have a witness and your son's fingerprints were found
on the stolen car that was used in the driveby
shooting. We cannot turn him loose in your custody.
This evening he will be taken to the district youth
correction center at Belview. Then in about two
weeks he will go before a judge. Since this is his first
arrest, the judge will probably sentence him to four
months of boot camp instead of him facing a jury trial
and receiving time in an adult prison. Come with me
Miss Allen, you will be allowed a thirty minute visit."

After Miss Allen left and all arrangements had
been made to transport Bruce Allen to Belview, Lt.
Elder decided to go home; he still had time to make it
to the Buieville High Tigers football game.

CHAPTER 6

Loco had enjoyed his breakfast and was sipping
on his coffee when Deacon Bines said, " Loco, for the
life of me I can't see how you can believe in God with
all of that stuff you be talking."

Possibly The Greatest Weight Control Breakthrough Of
The Century

After taking another sip of coffee Loco said,
"Deacon this may not answer your question, but this
is my basic outlook on the whole matter. I definitely
believe in one God, or a superior being.

"I believe our creator gave us a brain equipped
with reason and a logical thought process. This logic
and reasoning is a mental box that we can't get out
of. That is why we can't solve the old chicken and egg
riddle. That is why we believe there has to be a
beginning to everything no matter how far back.
From a scientific point of view there is no beginning or
ending because matter cannot be created or
destroyed, only changed from one form to another.
That says that what's here has always been here in
some form, but logically speaking that's impossible,
there has to be a higher level of reasoning ever u than
logic to ever understand our existence.

"Man made computers and designed them on the
binary base. It will never be able to count more than
one or two at a time. Electronically speaking #1 may
be a negative charge and #2 a positive charge. Then
when this process takes place at lightning speed you
have a super computer. Just like all computers are
limited to the binary design, man's reasoning is
limited to logic.

"Now, to change the subject, I'm going to speak
from a purely secular point of view on religions. The
invisible one God concept that is so reasonable that we
take for granted today has not always been the case.
In fact, almost all ancient civilizations had many gods
and goddesses. The three dominant early civilizations
of Egyptians, Greeks, and Romans all had many gods
And goddesses. Due to the Rosetta stone there is a
written history long before the invisible one God
concept. One of the early Egyptian Pharaohs was the
first to promote the invisible one God concept, but like
most things in ancient history, any new belief was
seen as a threat. In those days they had a simple
formula for dealing with threatening beliefs. Just kill
everyone with the belief. The established Egyptian

priests took that step, and thought that they had
wiped the invisible one God concept off of the face of
the earth forever. But, they were wrong, they didn't
get everyone, because centuries later the invisible one
God concept resurfaced full force among the Jews.

"Today the Jewish, Christian, and Moslem faiths
with their belief in one invisible God are by far the
dominant religions of the world. Not including the
Jewish and Moslem, there are over 2 billion Christians
alone world wide. Most other religions of the world
are mainly rules and guides for behavior and proper
living, but especially the Christian faith with its power
of the Holy Ghost, it really comes alive and stirs the
soul."

Rufus took his spiritual life very seriously.
Serving the Lord was a well established tradition in his
family. His uncle was a preacher, and his father was a
deacon. He also had a brother who was a minister
and two other brothers who were deacons.

Growing up, Rufus didn't have a choice about
going to church. His father's law was, "Me and my
family will serve the Lord." As a young man, Rufus had
sowed his share of wild oats, but even when young he
had the sense to never experiment with drugs.
Otherwise, he stayed out late, partied hard, and did a
lot of things he shouldn't have. Old Prospect Baptist
Church was the family church.

As young as he could remember as a boy, he had
sat in the pews of the Old Prospect Baptist Church.
While away in the navy he sort of backslid from his
religious upbringing. Even back home out of the navy
it was several years before he started back attending
church regularly. Then about ten years ago, he
became a deacon at Old Prospect Baptist Church. He
also has been a Sunday school teacher almost as long.

On Sunday mornings, Rufus liked for Janet to fix
him one of those old fashioned southern country

Possibly The Greatest Weight Control Breakthrough Of
The Century

breakfasts. She would fix homemade buttermilk
biscuits, smoked sausage, Canadian bacon, grits,
scrambled eggs, jelly, real butter, and orange juice.

After breakfast, they left for Sunday school.
Their regular pastor would not be preaching today.
Today's guest speaker would be visiting pastor Rev.
John B. Miley.

After the eleven o'clock service had started and
Rev. Miley launched into his sermon, Rufus' mind
drifted back to some of the great sermons his late
cousin Rev. Robert Flagler of Fernandina Beach Florida
used to preach. He remembered how Rev. Flagler
stressed Philippians fourth chapter, thirteen verse, "I
can do all things through Christ who strengthens me."
He stressed how anyone down and out with little or no
self confidence could repeat that verse over and over
to himself at least fifty times a day, and it would
guarantee him a successful life if only he kept saying
it.

Here is another good positive saying to repeat
fifty times or more each day to help one lose weight,
"I'm going to have a slim body, soon." The mind tries
to fulfill any image constantly presented to it. It
doesn't matter whether it is real or imagined, positive
or negative. The mind doesn't distinguish; it only
recognizes images. That is why it is so important to
think positively. That is why many of the old sayings
have grains of truth in them, sayings like, "Out of
sight out of mind," this can be a factor concerning sex
education, and a scary man can't win in gambling or
in battle.

The mind can't remember and deal with all of our
experiences at once, so it tends to remember and act
on the images that is presented the most constantly.
The images that are presented less and less will soon
be forgotten and not acted upon, but like in
everything there are exceptions. For instance, in
cases of trauma, an indelible imprint can be stamped
in one's memory in a matter of seconds and last
forever.

Possibly The Greatest Weight Control Breakthrough Of
The Century

Another old saying used when someone was
struggling with a problem was, "Go home and sleep
on it." There is great benefit in that because it allows
the subconscious mind time to help sort out and
organize the problem. The mind receives so many
conflicting images during a day that one would go
crazy if the mind didn't use sleeping and dreaming as
a sorting and filing process to organize recent images.
Most of us are not aware of the negative thought
images that we constantly feed our mind, but the
good thing is we can make a conscious effort to think
of positive images.

We have the ability to choose. One can decide
how he will treat another human being no matter how
that person treats him in return. The most powerful
positive thinking image I know of is to love and
forgive all people no matter how they treat you.

That doesn't mean you let anybody mistreat you.
You always defend yourself from attacks. You can
hate a person's ways and actions but still love the
person as a human being.

There may be cases when someone is
determined to make you hate him, then turn it over to
God, just repeat to yourself, " I can wish all people
goodwill, even if it's not returned." When you treat
other people well, and they don't return the favor, you
are not doing them a favor; you are doing yourself a
favor, because as long as you treat all not d people
well, you will stay a good person and mostly good
things will happen in your life. Then nothing nor
anybody can mentally defeat or destroy you.

You never see those who can genuinely love and
forgive in mental wards, you won't see them as bums
on the streets, or losers in any way. It is not enough
to say I don't hate anybody, what really matters is
how things are acted out. That means how you
actually treat all people on a day-to-day basis. There
is no way you can hate anybody, not even your enemy
if you make it a practice to treat all people well like
you would a loved one.

117

Possibly The Greatest Weight Control Breakthrough Of
The Century

Sure, there is a need for hate and all emotions,
but never hate anybody in your midst unless you are
prepared and able to destroy them, lest they destroy
you. The rule of thumb is to choose to treat all people
well with courtesy and respect. When Rev. Miley's
voice roared into one of those soul stirring hymns, it
brought Rufus' mind back to the present.

After the service, Rev. Miley stood at the front
door and shook the hands of the congregation as they
filed out. In the Towncar on their way to Mitchell's
Barbecue Restaurant for their Sunday dinner, Janet
asked Rufus how he liked the sermon Rev. Miley
preached.

"Rev. Miley preached a great sermon," said
Rufus, "but to be frank I spent most of the time
remembering some of the great sermons my late
cousin Robert Flagler used to preach. My view on
religion is I believe in God as much as anyone, but I
also believe God helps those who first help themselves.

"I believe if you do as good as you can do or go
as far as you can go, then some way, somehow God
will help you go the distance. Otherwise faith without
action is wasted."

They had a nice Sunday dinner of southern fried
chicken, barbecue ribs, mustard greens, potato salad,
macaroni and cheese, rice and gravy, sweet potato
pie, corn bread, and iced tea.

Once back home Rufus decided to send out
several queries to find a publisher for his almost
completed book.

Bruce Allen had never seen his mother as angry
and upset as when she found out he had not been
going to school. No matter how much he thought that
going to school was a waste of time, he knew he
didn't have any choice because his mother was dead
serious. The next day at school he felt out of place,

but he knew he had to make the best of a bad
situation.

Somehow, he got through his first day back.

He felt especially elated when the bell ring ended
the school day. Not so much because school was
letting out but because he was going to see LaTonya.
He and LaTonya were watching TV when they heard
someone knocking on her front door.

When Bruce heard someone ask for him with an
unmistaken tone of authority, he knew instantly it was
the police and he knew why they were there.

He knew it was too late to go out the back door
because they had already seen him sitting on the
couch. He knew there was no point in trying to resist,
he might as well go quietly.

After being arrested and taken to the station, he
was fingerprinted and booked. During questioning, he
denied having anything to do with any driveby
shooting. They claimed they lifted his fingerprints off
of a gray Honda Accord that had been stolen the night
of the driveby shooting.

Lt. Elder repeatedly asked him if he was in
anyway involved in a driveby shooting. Each time
they asked, he denied everything. Later, what
bothered him most was the pain and hurt in his
mother's eyes. He felt he had truly let his mother
down. He loved his mother more than life itself. He
decided then and there that if he ever got through this
trouble he would swear before God to go straight,
because never again would he put his mother through
that kind of hurt and pain.

After he had told his mother how sorry he was
for having hurt her, he then told her if the Lord got
him through this, he would finish school and leave
gangs and drugs behind. With tears in his eyes, he
told his mother good by. Sergeant Victory Kocher, a
young detective on the night shift, transported him
the thirty miles to the district youth correction center
at ht shi Belview.

Possibly The Greatest Weight Control Breakthrough Of
The Century

At the center he was issued brogans, coveralls,
underwear, tooth paste and tooth brush, and bed
linen. The next morning he had to meet with the
center's chief psychiatrist Doctor Zebedee Moore, then
he had an appointment with the center's rehabilitated
strong man, Chaplain David Taylor. He was assigned
to dormitory "B." Each dorm was managed by a
supervisor.

He was to report to his dorm supervisor any
problems or criticism he had. He was told he would
be there until his court date in about two weeks.
Bruce was not used to being told everything to do, in
fact he had never had any strict discipline, period. He
managed to adjust to the regimental style of life
better than he at first imagined. He had been at the
center now for almost two weeks, and his court date
would be coming up in a few days.

It's been almost two weeks now since Lt. Elder
put those youth gang leaders behind bars. Rufus felt
good about how his life was going at the present.
Business was good at the restaurant. The gang
problem had been taken care of. He had found a
publisher for his book. So he decided he would
celebrate by buying Janet a diamond ring.

Lee's Press, Inc. a small publishing company
would be publishing his first book. The small
publishing company couldn't promote it as much as
Rufus knew it deserved, so he knew if the book was
going to make it big he would have to do a lot of the
promoting himself. He would try to get on the Frances
Waddell talk show and as many talk shows as possible.

The publishing company was going to start off
with sixty thousand copies for the first printing. They
will give him two hundred copies to give to friends, do
self-promoting, sell or do as he pleased. The
publisher was going to run some ads in a few big city
newspapers, but Rufus knew that for the book to sell

he would have to make the rounds of talk shows and
hustle his own book.

Juvenile Judge Fred Smith had very little
sympathy for spoiled, ill-raised, undisciplined
youngsters. He felt lack of discipline was the root
cause of all the problems with today's youths. Most of
the kids that come before him have never been
conditioned to fear punishment or consequences.
Many of these kids have never heard a cold hard firm
voice of authority demanding obedience. They look at
him wide-eyed and bewildered when he chews them
out.

Judge Smith knew that most of the kids that
come before him would never be there if someone
would have shown them love and put the fear of
punishment and consequences in them the first time
they broke the law. Most of the people running
around talking about people being mean spirited are
too shallow to see past their noses. They are
hollering that conservatives don't have any
compassion. They don't know what real compassion
is. Real compassion is about protecting and saving
the whole country, not about saving a few and letting
the whole country perish and go to hell.

We all have a free will to adapt, but to waste
compassion on those that choose not to adapt is not
only a waste of time, it is dangerous. All animal or
specie survival is dependent on their ability to adapt
to their environment, otherwise they perish. Not
forcing people to depend on themselves, their family,
their extended family, their community, and private
organizations is being weak, irresponsible, and
negligent, not showing compassion.

It is always easier to be weak and take the
course of least resistance, but in the end it will cost
this country dearly if not destroy it. Real compassion
is to be prepared to survive as an organized society

under all conditions, even if the government goes broke and money becomes worthless. Trying to get liberals to understand that is like talking to a brick wall.

Those with the foresight and wisdom must speak out on the necessity of conditioning people to depend on each other as much as possible for their survival. No one knows how much time we have to prepare, but the destruction of moral and family values are always the last stage. Big government is the cause of the problem, not the answer.

Judge Smith knew he could save more of these youngsters if he could put the fear of God in them, thereby conditioning them to fear punishment and consequences.

Bruce didn't know what to expect as he sat in juvenile court that Monday morning when his name was called. His mother was sitting on his left, and uniformed officer Corporal Andrew Desantis was on his right. After his name was called, Officer Desantis escorted him to a rail about ten feet in front of the judge then left him alone and stood off to one side.

As Bruce stood there, the judge continued to read a report.

"State your name," said Judge Smith to Bruce in a loud, demanding voice.

"Bruce Allen, your honor" (as he had been coached).

"How do you plead to the charges?" said Judge Smith.

"Not guilty, your honor."

"We have an eye witness, and how did your fingerprints get on a stolen car that was believed to be used in the driveby shooting?"

"I don't know, your honor."

"Young man, you could go before a jury and be sentenced to several years of hard time in prison as an

adult, but since this is the first time you have come
before me, I am going to sentence you to four months
of boot camp at Pine Valley Youth Correction
Institution. But if you ever come before me again,
young man you are going to be put away for a long,
long time. Do you hear me young man?" said Judge
Smith in a loud cold angry voice.

"Yes sir, your honor."

"Take him away, bailiff," said Judge Smith.

Bruce was allowed to say good bye to his mother
and LaTonya. Then he was taken to boot camp at Pine
Valley Correction Institution.

At Pine Valley everything was done in regimental
style like in a real military boot camp. After arriving
at Pine Valley, he was issued clothing and assigned a
bunk in an open bay dormitory. Every morning they
had to get up at five thirty.

They were given thirty minutes to make their
beds with perfect hospital corners, brush their teeth,
shave, shower, etc.. Breakfast was served from six to
seven.

Calisthenics was from seven to nine. Classes
and training were from nine to twelve. Lunch from
twelve to one. Classes and training from one to four
thirty. Dinner from four thirty to five thirty.
Recreation and leisure time from five thirty to ten
p.m.. At ten p.m. all lights out. Bruce was taught to
say yes sir or no sir to every command or instruction.
Some of the training instructors were retired military.

One of his instructors was a mean, tough,
computer whiz named Sergeant Johnnie Roberson.
Bruce remembers his first morning at reveille. They
had to stand at attention while Sergeant Roberson
walked up and down the line inspecting the prisoners.
He stopped in front of Bruce and placed his face about
four inches from his. "What is your name prisoner?"
said Sergeant Roberson in a loud, angry voice.

"Bruce Allen, sir."

"I can't hear you."

"Bruce Allen, sir," said he in a loud voice.

Possibly The Greatest Weight Control Breakthrough Of
The Century

"I still can't hear you."

"Bruce Allen, sir," said he almost yelling.

"Where you from prisoner?"

"Buieville, Georgia, sir."

"The only thing that comes from there is skunks and punks, which one are you prisoner?"

"Neither, sir."

"Are you calling me a liar prisoner?"

"No sir."

"I'm going to be watching you prisoner, and if I see you step out of line, your ass is grass and I'm the lawn mower, do you hear me prisoner?"

"Yes sir."

Sergeant Roberson took several steps backward, then he yelled out, "Column right, hut, two, three, four, hut, two, three, four," and on they marched to the dining hall.

At first, Bruce wanted to rebel and resist being told everything to do, but after a while he learned to control his anger and actions. Then for the first time in his life he felt a new power and control over his actions. He realized one's own actions determines the results one gets out of life. After more than a month at Pine Valley, Bruce knew that he was going to make it. He had gained enough self-control to do the right thing and stay out of trouble.

His mother and LaTonya visited and stood by him. The least he could do would be to stay out of trouble and not let them down.

CHAPTER 7

It's been almost a week since Rufus received his free two hundred copies of his first book, "Why We Must Dismantle The Welfare State By Rufus Thomas." Rufus had immediately started doing his share to promote his new book. He sent copies to all of the major book suppliers around the country.

Possibly The Greatest Weight Control Breakthrough Of
The Century

He sent copies to all of the largest big city
newspapers. He also sent copies to major public and
college library systems around the country.

He requested to be on several talk shows. He
offered to lecture and sign copies of his book at public
functions, churches, prisons, etc. Within the next
three months, he had invitations to appear on the
Frances Waddell talk show and several other talk
shows. Next month he was scheduled to speak at
Pine Valley Youth Correction Institution.

Rufus had no intention of ever seeking public
office himself, but if he could convince just one person
in office of the dangers of big government and the
welfare state, that alone would make it all worthwhile.
The government has taken on a provider role and is
saddled with huge financial burdens with millions and
millions of people, some totally dependent on the
government for their only survival. That is
irresponsible and negligent for any free society to do,
especially when the government doesn't have the self-
discipline to control spending. What are all those
people to do when the government goes broke? Only
a fool will believe it can't happen.

It is obvious that it is only a matter of time
before the debt gets so big the government can't raise
taxes high enough, borrow enough money, or sell
enough bonds to finance it.

Then the government won't have any choice but
to print more and more money. After a while printing
all of this money will cause hyper-inflation making the
greenback practically worthless. With a very weak
nuclear family and extended family system, this
country could lose fifty million plus people and split
along regional and ethnic lines. With our loose family
and moral values, there is no solid foundation left to
organize and rebuild upon. With money being
worthless, there would be nothing the government
could do without international help.

But if the dollar went down, it would probably
bring the world economy down with it. The economy

is already so distorted that our currency is like
Monopoly money with the way sports figures and
entertainers are being paid.

What are we to do, with the family and the
extended family structure almost destroyed from fifty
years of becoming dependent on an over generous,
non-disciplining, and super rich sugar daddy
government. On the other hand, when responsibility
is passed to the states and local governments that
should help rebuild the family foundation, then if the
central government went broke, all would not be lost.

One month later Rufus was up, up, thirty three
thousand feet into "The long, delirious burning blue,"
The wild blue yonder, "Where never lark, or even
eagle flew," on his way to the Big Apple to appear on
the Frances Waddell talk show. It was an all expense
paid trip.

On the show, Rufus was asked how can you be
so uncaring as to cut out school children's lunch
program money?

"We have to ask ourselves this question," said
Rufus,

"which is more important, to cause much
hardship or lose the whole country? I say save the
country first, then the children may have to take a
lunch pail or bag to school or whatever is necessary.
People will always find a way to survive on their own
unless they depend on the government so long and
forget how to do for themselves."

After returning to Buieville, Rufus enjoyed his
new fame.

He and his book received a big write up in the
"Buieville Daily Times." His publisher reported that his
book was selling great.

At the rate they were selling, the initial sixty
thousand would be sold out in two weeks. The
publisher was already making preparations for a
second printing.

Three weeks later Rufus spoke at Pine Valley
Youth Correction Institution. Afterward he signed

126

copies of his new book. As Rufus was signing books
he was surprised and taken aback when Bruce Allen
wanted Rufus to sign a book for him.

Rufus thought of his religious upbringing, he
thought of a youth gone astray, and he thought of the
power of forgiveness.

Rufus stared at the young man.

"Mr. Thomas," said Bruce Allen, "I'm sure you
know who I am."

"I do?"

"If you find it in your heart to forgive me of the
wrong I've done you, I just want you to know that I'm
truly sorry."

"What are you going to do when you get out?"
said Rufus.

"I promised my mom that I would finish school,
sir."

Rufus thought that a young man living with his
family in the Jimmy Carroll Housing Projects could use
some pocket spending money. "I'll tell you what
young man, if you are willing to work, come to see me
at the restaurant when you get out." That night Rufus
lay relaxing in bed after he and Janet had made love.
"You know Janet," said Rufus "a strange thing
happened to me today at my speaking engagement at
Pine Valley Correction Institution. One of the youths
convicted in the driveby shooting on my restaurant
bought one of my books and wanted me to sign it. He
told me he was sorry about what he had done. I not
only autographed his book, I offered him a job when
he gets out, but I can't help but wonder if I did a
dumb thing."

"Honey, you've always enjoyed helping people.
You wouldn't be happy any other way."

"I guess you're right, dear. Good night, darling,"
said Rufus.

After four months, Bruce had done his time and
was let out of boot camp, but he still was on

probation for another four years. Bruce was determined to keep his promise to his mom.

He decided to stay away from his old friends and the gang. He decided no matter what, he was going to finish school. He got word that Boom Boom had become leader of the Young Vipers. Bruce tried out for the Buieville High basketball team.

He not only made the team, he was going to be a starter.

His girl friend LaTonya had passed her high school G.E.D. and was scheduled to enroll at Buieville Community College the next quarter to get her L.P.N. degree. Three weeks later, Bruce and LaTonya were watching TV when the newscaster reported that a local gang leader who went by the name of Boom Boom was killed last night in a driveby shooting.

A few nights later Bruce was sitting with LaTonya on the sofa. "You know, LaTonya," said Bruce, "I stopped by the funeral home this afternoon to see Boom Boom, and deep down in my soul, I knew that the body lying there could just as easily have been me. Truly the Lord does work in mysterious ways," said Bruce. "At the time I thought being arrested was the worst thing that could have happened to me, but as it turned out being arrested and going to boot camp was actually the very best thing to ever happen to me. It gave me a second chance to live, and I'm going to make the best of it. Boom Boom blew his second chance, but not me."

"Honey, I am so proud of you," said LaTonya.

"Thank you dear, but I could never have done it without you and mom's support."

Rufus was back in the kitchen when Erica stuck her head in the doorway. "Mr. Thomas, there is a young man out here that says he would like to talk with you."

"Erica, tell him I'll be there in a minute." As Rufus pushed open the kitchen door he recognized the young man as Bruce Allen immediately. Rufus walked

behind the counter to right across from where Bruce
Allen was standing.

"Hello, Mr. Thomas," said Bruce Allen as Rufus
came to a stop.

"Hello Bruce."

"Mr. Thomas, I came by to see if you are still
willing to give me a job."

" We close around three thirty during the week,
but we stay open to nine p.m. on Friday and
Saturdays, so I can let you come in for a twelve hour
day on Saturday if you would like that."

"Yes sir, Mr. Thomas. I certainly would
appreciate it."

"When would you like to start?"

"Quick as I can; this Saturday will be fine."

"Fine," said Rufus, "I will pay you minimum
wage; be here at eight a.m. this Saturday."

"Yes sir, I'll be here, and thank you very much
Mr. Thomas."

Rufus knew about fifty dollars wasn't a lot of
money, but it would help teach the youth the work
ethic and provide him with pocket money. After four
Saturdays Bruce proved to be a dependable, willing
worker. Rufus and Bruce sort of took to each other.
Rufus never had a son and Bruce never had a dad; it
seemed to be a perfect match. Already, Rufus had
taken Bruce fishing in his boat, the first time Bruce had
ever been fishing in his life.

Rufus hadn't seen Loco in quite a while, but
sooner or later he always comes around. Detective
Marvin Elder stopped by the restaurant often to chat a
few minutes and have a cup of coffee with Rufus.
Rufus' book had gone into its second printing. He
couldn't judge how much effect his book had to do
with the mood of the country, but he took comfort in
observing the whole country going through a peaceful
revolution. Even the bleeding heart liberals were
admitting something had to be done about the welfare
mess. Only in the U.S.A. can a poor shy country boy

Possibly The Greatest Weight Control Breakthrough Of
The Century

rise up and touch the heartbeat of America. Rufus decided to end his book by saying, God bless America.

THE END

FREDDIE L. SIRMANS, SR.
Self Made
Writer/Publisher/Philosopher/Inventor

WEBSITE: FLSirmans.com